# The Complete William Kelley Program
## From Past to Present

Dr Eric Wood, ND, MA

with Pamela McDougle, NC

The Complete William Kelley Program From Past to Present



Printed by B.C. Allen Publishing and Tonic Books
144 N 7th St. #525
Brooklyn, NY 11249

Now taking manuscript submissions and book ideas at any stage of the process: submissions@tonicbooks.online

Printed in the United States of America

Editor: Krista Munster
Interior Design: Susan Veach

ISBN: 979-8-9857517-9-6  (Paperback)

## Pamela McDougle's Background as a Nutritionist

Pamela McDougle spent seven years with the late Dr. William Donald Kelley, an orthodontist, who helped himself survive pancreatic cancer with a unique cancer protocol using high potency proteolytic enzymes from 40 to 72 capsules daily. She has been in practice for over thirty years and has seen about 5,000 patients. As a nutritionist, she also has a background of training in raw food nutrition with the Ann Wigmore Institute, formerly in Boston, Massachusetts.

Her counterpart was the late Dr. Nicholas Gonzalez, M.D., who also trained with Dr. Kelley and was the protégé of the late Dr. Robert Good, M.D., PhD., immunologist, president, and director of Sloan-Kettering Hospital, an institution in New York City. With higher visibility, Dr. Gonzalez had a large clinical practice and received a $1.4 million grant from the NIH Complementary Alternative Medicine branch and worked with Columbia Medical Institute to document clinical pancreatic cancer patients using traditional and the proteolytic enzyme protocol. The study was biased, and because of this, the results showed a survival of 14 months with traditional therapy and 4 months with the proteolytic enzyme treatment.

I have known and worked with Pamela McDougle for over 20 years and have seen some remarkable results when traditional therapy failed.

### The Book

This book is a guide to using systemic enzyme therapy specifically for cancer. The first part deals with detoxification of "Body Burdens," such as organic and inorganic toxic accumulations, and viral, bacterial, and fungal mold infections, and with cleansing detoxification procedures using the three largest surface area organs—the gastrointestinal tract, the liver, and the skin—as the fastest way to eliminate burdens so the body can save its resources to address the main problem—cancer.

The later chapters focus on the use of a large number of digestive enzymes, from 40 to 72 capsules per day, with added extra bovine Chymotrypsin in their high potency enzymes. Though these enzymes are used when not eating, Pamela and Dr. Wood tell me that the use of enzymes capsules during a meal also aids in the process. The authors strictly adhere to the recommendation of the five-day (5) periods off all enzymes every 25 days as mandatory for the enzyme therapy success.

**Kurt Isselbacher, MD, PhD of Harvard**


Most of my colleagues have always been skeptical that digestive enzymes, which are macromolecules, could even cross the gastrointestinal barrier, let alone their systemic therapeutic effects. I point out to them that the landmark basic science research was done on macromolecules crossing the intestinal barrier by one of the greatest physician researchers, the late Kurt Isselbacher, MD. He was a German immigrant born of Jewish decent and became Professor of Medicine at Harvard Medical School and the director of Massachusetts General Hospital, focusing on the gastrointestinal system, and co-editor of the first editions of Harrison's Textbook of Medicine. Isselbacher and Alan Walker studied the passage of the macromolecule Horse radish Peroxidase enzyme from the gastrointestinal tract to the mesenteric lymph system, then to the liver portal blood (Walker A, Isselbacher KJ Lab. Investigation Vol25, 6, 675, 1971; *Gastroenterology* 67:531–550, 1974; *Journal of Immunology* Vol. 115, 3, 1975). They found these large molecules could cross over into the mesentery lymphatic and blood circulatory systems.

## My Experience with Enzyme Therapy in Post-Operative Patients of Thirty-Seven Years

On a practical level, the research above was applicable to patient management. As a urological cancer and reconstructive surgeon for thirty-seven years, our surgery often involved organ and cancer resection and reconstruction of a new bladder reservoir using intestinal tracts. The surgery often required five hours or longer, with massive soft tissue and muscle debris and ecchymoses in the post-operative period. I learned from the plastic surgeons to use protease enzymes orally to clear up the massive debris inside the body and on skin surfaces with ecchymoses and hematomas by its digestion of necrotic tissues, which cleared up within five to 7 days. With or without the science above, I knew these macromolecules could cross the intestinal barrier and digest all the debris in the blood and adjacent to organs after surgery.

## Digestive and Systemic Use of Digestive Enzymes Worldwide

In the 1950s to 1970s, the closest American exposure to use of digestive enzymes commercially was "Adolf's meat tenderizer," which contains Bromelain enzymes from pineapple stems and works beautifully to predigest and soften meats.

Having lectured in Europe and Japan in the past, I observed that their use of enzymes is not only for digestion and flavoring but also systemically for pain relief like aspirin, as an anti-inflammatory drug like steroids, and as an antidote for mild food allergies. It is regarded as a form of medication and the largest, most reputable company often stemmed from pharmaceutical companies such as Amano, Shin Nihon Chemicals (Japan) and formally Danisco (Dan- mark sold to Dupont USA). Most of the enzymes in Japan originate as by-products of Aspergillus Oryzae, Sojae, etc. and other funguses (saprotrophic). They differ from human and animal enzymes as they function at a wide pH range, from 2 to 10, whereas human and animal enzymes function mostly at a pH of 7–8. Amano has researched over 4,000 enzymes ranging from digestion to health uses, such as collagenase, and as industrial enzymes. So internationally, the digestive and health use of enzymes is not foreign as in the United States. Enzymes generally are catalysts for most metabolic processes and known worldwide as a simple method for fermentation or "pre digestion" of any protein, fats, and sugars.

I believe that, rather than a direct attack on the cancer cell itself, the use of the proteolytic systemic enzyme therapy for cancers is a form of "immunotherapy," addressing the "Transforming Growth Factor beta (TGF $B$)" pathway, which can neutralize its immune suppressive lymphocytes and neutrophils, etc. TGF $B$ Pleiotropic cytokine is often elevated in cancer patients, and it can promote immunosuppression signaling via blocking T cell Natural killer cell (NK), CD8+

*cytotoxic* T cells (CTL), Lymphokine-activated Killer cells, and the Tregs system, which promotes cancer invasion and metastasis at the cancer microenvironment level.

Alpha 2 Macroglobulin (alpha 2 M) can neutralize TGF B immune suppression by binding with a proteolytic enzyme (TGF- Macroglobulin-Protease) or by another method using Methylamine and a complex forming with (TGF *B*–Macroglobulin-Methylamine). The two (2) above activated complexes neutralize TGF *B* immune suppression and allow the NK cells, CTL cells, (LAK) Lymphokine-activated Killer cells, etc. to attack and kill the cancer cells (Harthun NL, Slingluff CL J. *Immunotherapy* 21(2), 85–94, 1998).

**The future of newer molecules in basic and clinical investigation, such as Galunisertib kinase inhibitor, may function similarly as Proteolytic Enzymes-Alpha 2 Macroglobulin complex on Transforming Growth Factor *B*.**

As proteolytic enzymes bind with the alpha 2 Macroglobulin forming a TGF *b*-Macroglobulin-Protease complex, we now have a new smaller molecule in investigation, such as Galunisertib kinase inhibitor, which can neutralize and bind with the TGF *b*.

From 2015 through 2018, it's been shown that newer molecules such as Galunisertib-TGF *b* complex can also neutralize the TGF *b* Immune suppressive effects. Galunisertib (TGF beta receptor I) kinase inhibitor has been studied as a single agent as well as in a combination approach with an additional PD-L1 immunotherapy and has shown remarkable complete response in colon cancer models. Alone, Galunisertib has an inhibitor memory on animal cancer studies, but combining Galunisertib with a another PD1 inhibitor / PD-L1 checkpoint inhibitors (nivolumab and durvalumab) has a synergistic effect (Holmgaard RB, J. *Immunotherapy of Cancer* 6:47, 2018).

Enzymes bind with alpha 2 Macroglobulin to neutralize the bad effects of overproduction of TGF *B*, Transforming Growth Factors *B*. With time and further research, there will be newer molecules that will neutralize the immunosuppressive effects of TGF *b*.

We even have a recent publication from the University of Nebraska Medical showing that for metastatic prostatic cancer to the bones, the use of Bipolar androgen therapy (BAT) allows testosterone to prime up polymorphonuclear neutrophils by altering TGF *b* receptor and allow anti-tumor immune response in metastatic bone lesions (Alsamraae M, Cook LM. Androgen-mediated TGF Expression suppresses anti-tumor neutrophil response in bone metastatic prostate cancer. December 31, 2022).

## Other Degradation of Systemic Foreign Protein in Our Bodies with the Use of Enzymes

More recently, world news shows the effectiveness of enzymes to digest abnormal proteins in the body. It is well known that the new form of vaccines is not like the old fashioned "attenuated virus" but are mRNA vaccines such as the COVID 19 mRNA Vaccine, with an unexpected byproduct called a "Spike Protein" of SARS-CoV-2 in our blood. This new protein cannot be destroyed easily and may be related to some clinical complications such as myocarditis of the heart.

Dr. Peter McCullough has been the biggest advocate to caution all of us to the mRNA vaccine and its potential dangerous adverse effects. Two scientific publications have shown that Bromelain enzyme from pineapple stem and natto kinase enzyme (a Japanese fermented soy product from Bacillus subtilis) can degrade this Spike Protein from our blood (Yonker LM, *Circulation* 47:867, 2023; Tanikkawa, T., *Molecule* 202,27, 5405). Again, the use of natural enzymes has wide implications and applications with minimal adverse effects may have use in clinical medicine other than for cancer support.

**There is more research to be done to build on our understanding of the role of proteolytic enzymes in immune function and disease.**

The work of Dr. William Kelley, Dr. Nicholas Gonzales, and Pamela McDougle was a phenomenon without a clear scientific rationale at that time. In more recent years, we have the landmark discoveries b Nobel Prize winners James Allison (USA) of CTLA-4 protein on immune cells and Tasuku Honjo (Japan) of cell death 1 PD-1 protein again on immune cells that were defective or "T cell brake." The evolution of immune cancer treatments focused on the immune cells rather than the cancer cells has changed clinical cancer treatment forever! We are now focused on how to release the anti-cancer immune response by monoclonal antibodies inhibitors to block the new protein mutations.

Could it be that the proteolytic enzymes also can recognize abnormal new proteins from mutations on cancer cells and on immune cells? Could these enzymes indiscriminately digest any new protein mutations on cell surfaces and on necrotic cancer cell fragments in the body circulation?

In addition, the final Total Cancer Genome Atlas in 33 cancers (TCGA) also identified new mutations producing new proteins on cancer surface and in the cytoplasm, which has led to "targeted therapy" using monoclonal antibodies and smaller molecules to bind with all new mutations. Could it be that the proteolytic enzymes recognize new mutated proteins on and in cancers and in necrotic fragments of cancers in blood and can digest foreign cancer proteins?

**Must Read for All!**

I recommend people read this book and share it with their medical doctors to better understand an age-old systemic protease enzyme therapy in cancer diseases.

We look forward to the future medical science developments after you finish reading the book.

**George Yu M.D. October 30, 2023, YuFoundation.org**


In this new book, Dr. Wood introduces the traditional naturopathic concept of addressing the terrain and not solely the lesion or microbe in isolation, and he does so in a compellingly well-articulated and biologically comprehensive manner. He addresses the many factors that are injuring the health of people, from contaminated food and pervasive mold and mycotoxins to extreme stress. This is a truly naturopathic approach, with a basis in addressing the disturbances to the determinants of health, coupled with comprehensive intake, including laboratory tests. A holistic approach to therapy and a clearly mapped out regimen follows. This book is clearly the reflection of years of deep study and practice—our profession needs more like it.

**Fraser Smith, MATD, ND**

**Professor**

**Assistant Dean for Naturopathic Medicine,**

**College of Professional Studies**

**National University of Health Sciences**


Dr. Wood brings clarity to one of the most pressing issues of our day: not only has cancer risen in the past 100 years to become the #2 cause of death right after heart disease, but cancer incidence in people younger than 50 is now on the rise as well.

Eric Wood recognizes that while cancer is a multifactorial disease, key contributors still unacknowledged today by the conventional medical model include the pernicious influence of the exposome, all of the non-genetic factors that coalesce into the disease we call cancer. Indeed, 90–95% of cancer has its roots in environmental factors: diet, environmental pollution, and lifestyle.

Dr Wood brilliantly analyzes the pivotal work of Dr William Kelley in successfully working with cancer and updates this approach so that it fits into the 21st century framework, which encompasses the always evolving science of medicine and increasing awareness of the impact of environmental chemicals on cancer initiation and progression.

If you are faced with a diagnosis of cancer and are

seeking strategies for care, this book will help you understand the history and clinical use of pancreatic proteolytic enzymes in cancer.

**Anne Marie Fine, NMD,**

**FAAEM Medical Director**

**Environmental Medicine Education International, LLC**

**Fellow, American Academy of Environmental Medicine**


I first met Pamela about twenty years ago when she came into my office for a consultation. At that time, she was gaining expertise from Dr William Kelley on his cancer protocols and helping him to update and improve them. I had gotten my cancer education from Dr. Donato Garcia, and we were doing IPT Low dose chemotherapy and other supportive integrative cancer therapies. After meeting Pamela, I read all I could about Dr. Kelley and his methods, and we had many long conversations about which methods worked the best. Our back-and-forth dialogues were very educational for both of us, and we learned much from each other.

As time went along, Pamela would refer me some of her most complicated patients so we could help tune them up medically and I would send them back to her with little hope that they would survive.

Amazingly, many of them did.

While Pamela was using the methods described in this book, she also had a keen insight into the mental emotional condition of her patients. We would often discuss this. It was hard for me to believe at the time that the enzymes, diet, and sauna could cause a remission in a Stage IV cancer patient who had already failed conventional and other treatments.

I kept asking her, "There must be more to this. What else are you doing?  What is your secret?"

Finally, after quite a lot of probing, she said, "After doing an initial intake, I would say to them, 'Why do you think you got this cancer? Do you have any idea?' Almost every person would tell me what was stressing them that they believed caused the cancer: relationships with spouses and children, their jobs, etc. After listening to them, I would very quietly say to them (holding them in the space of love), 'Do you have a plan for how you are going to resolve these issues?' I would try to guide them, without pressure, to explore this. I always suspected that there were unconscious reasons as well, and some patients found modalities that would help them explore this."

During their once-a-week sessions with Pamela, at the end she would gently ask them, "How is the plan going (or have you developed a plan) to address the stressors in your life?" She never ventured to give them the answers. She knew that someone would never consciously do this to themselves, but it might be a decision they made at some point and were unaware of it. "They have the answers, I just had to get them to look and see and, if true, to find them." She said, "When they did, they would have a tremendous 'Aha!' moment and they would start to get better.

I found this remarkable.

Another very important factor of her insights into helping her patients was their malnutrition. Pamela discovered many had extreme amino acid deficiency, resulting in severe protein malnutrition. They had very low serum albumin, low hemoglobin, and other very decreased immune factors. When she first brought this to my attention, I told her about a product that my company, Body Health, was manufacturing called Perfect Amino. It is a blend of eight essential amino acids that is the most effective product to improve protein synthesis. She found that giving them high doses of Perfect Amino allowed her patients to regain their immune health, improve their anemias, give them energy, and improve their mental outlook. She had one very severe case with an upper intestinal cancer who could not eat enough protein to survive. Pamela decided to give them Perfect Amino retention enemas and with the extra amino acids coming in, after months of this therapy the patient improved and their blood protein levels normalized. **The key to Pamela's success seems to be combining all these elements together: enzymes, diet, sauna, nutritional and herbal supplements, and psychological/emotional exploration and support.**

Once Pamela had refined her methods, she began teaching them to physicians and nutritionists who wanted to treat cancer. Many took advantage of her expertise and experience, and she recruited me to teach the groups of doctors about amino acid therapy in cancer patients. We taught hundreds of physicians her techniques to the betterment of many.

Pamela in her **modesty** will not tell you this, but she is one of the most remarkable women to have impacted health care. While not formally trained in oncology medicine, her curiosity to explore, test, and refine in order to do the best for her patients is compelling. She studied many enzyme varieties and worked with manufacturers to make sure she had the best ones. Same with probiotics and various herb and mushroom varieties; she worked to figure out what were the best remedies for intestinal dysbiosis, and of course, what were the best amino acids, all while being a busy wife, mother, and grandmother. Pamela is a pioneer and on her own is making a great impact, helping sick cancer patients have a better and longer life.

This book is a testament to the science and art of cancer care that she has uncovered.

I know, given her drive and enthusiasm for learning and exploration, that it's only a summary of what she has learned up to this point. I am sure in another few years there will be more insights and truths revealed.

Pamela, my friend, well done on this wonderful work. You have helped so many and so are loved by many. Thank you for your dedication to humanity. You are a giant in the helping profession. God Bless.

**David Minkoff, MD**

**Lifeworks Wellness Center, Clearwater, Florida**

# OUTLINE

# DEDICATION AND THANKS

*We would like to take this opportunity to dedicate this work to Dr. William Kelley, whose pioneering efforts not only saved his life but have helped countless others battling cancer.*

***

A big thank you goes to Pamela McDougle for continuing Kelley's legacy in working with thousands of clients and training many practitioners in this novel approach over the last 25+ years.

In memory of Terry W., whose light left us too early.

Finally, Dr. Wood would like to thank his daughter Sofie Annelise and all the children of the world for inspiring him to try and make the world a healthier place.

# INTRODUCTION:

## Why the Need for an Updated Program and Our Connection to This Work

Dr. Eric Wood, ND, MA and Pamela McDougle, NC

NOTE: We highly suggest that anyone contemplating implementing this program read the ENTIRE book before beginning any part of the program for many reasons, including safety.

### A Brief Historical Background on the Protocol

William Kelley never began his career intending to work primarily with cancer patients. He was a Texas dentist by training, and until his own life-changing diagnosis of pancreatic cancer in the early 1960s, that is what his life's work was focused on. But life has a funny way of getting in the way when we're making other plans, as the saying goes. And as for Dr. Kelley, this certainly seems to be the case. Given next to no chance or hope of long-term survival by his then doctors, Dr. Kelley went through what many people do when they're given a "terminal diagnosis": a personal crisis. However, this crisis quickly turned to action, and Kelley's energies were fervently directed at saving his own life. Benefitting from his medical training and ability to research, he quickly began to delve into medical annals, going back all the way to the late 1800s and early 1900s. In this process, he discovered the little-known and oft-forgotten work of predecessor physicians and scientists such as John Beard, who had brought forth groundbreaking ideas and theories surrounding cancer and enzymes and thoughts on how cancer could be differently and perhaps more effectively addressed. The results of this mission became eventually codified into what we now term "the Kelley protocol"—his own ad hoc, scientifically-based but anecdotally chronicled set of holistic interventions, including particular dietary guidelines, "metabolic testing," detoxification therapies, and perhaps most importantly, the use of pancreatic enzymes as a cornerstone of his own "protocol."

His own results, on some level, speak for themselves: Dr. Kelley survived his immediate health crisis and gradually was able to stabilize his health and return to medical practice and lived for another forty-plus years. Due to his life-changing event and the fact that word started to get out that he had survived this so-often fatal diagnosis, he began to attract patients who wondered if he could help them. Remember, this was the 1960s, and there were considerably even fewer options for cancer care (conventional or "alternative") back then than there are now. Dr. Kelley began to work with individuals who had been given little to no hope for recovery and was astonishingly able to help many, many individuals who were otherwise written off. Pamela McDougle witnessed this firsthand, working by his side in clinical practice for approximately seven years in the 1990s. Initially, he worked in Texas and then later in Washington State.

However, the Kelley protocol, like any good protocol, was not a *"static entity"* for decades on end. As times changed, functional and integrative medicine testing became available, and perhaps most crucially, as people's health needs and statuses changed, the program evolved as well. What Dr. Kelley practiced in the 1960s and 70s *NEEDED* to evolve because, frankly, on average, the overall vitality and health of most people have been diminishing since that time on many levels (at least in North America). This is for many reasons, but some of the primary ones include poor nutritional intakes, the introduction of more pesticides and genetically modified foods, decreasing amounts of sleep, increasingly busy and stressful lives, growing numbers and types of diverse environmental toxicants (including electromagnetic fields from all kinds of electronic devices), and more. We simply, on average, have more health threats to contend with than we did in the 1960s and 70s and have more demanding lifestyles that allow for less rest and recuperation.

Pamela McDougle, a contributor to this book and my mentor in this area of work, was herself Dr. Kelley's last student mentor. As mentioned, she trained and worked with Dr. William Kelley for seven years by his side in the 1990s as a trained nutritional consultant. And month after month, they chronicled cases, reviewing what seemed to work well and what didn't, and theorized what could be done differently or better as enough trends made themselves apparent in the accumulating cases in conjunction with scouring extant medical literature. This ultimately resulted in evolving the program in many ways, including adding particular functional medicine tests, new dietary guidelines to reflect what seemed to work best for the vast majority of clients, customized pancreatic enzymes to a potency and composition blend not otherwise commercially available, specified sauna and other forms of detoxification guidelines to work more effectively and profoundly, and more. Like all conscientious, science-minded practitioners, they kept meticulous records of these cases to allow for later review to look for positive and negative trends regarding outcomes to further refine prescriptive guidelines that were being given to clients of all kinds of cancer.

Good clinicians and scientists never "rest on their laurels" if something isn't working well, and as time progressed into the 1980s and especially the 1990s, it was becoming apparent to Dr. Kelley that the program had to evolve as he wasn't continuing to get the degree of success as he did years earlier. Thus, with Ms. McDougle's help, the program became more comprehensive and encompassing of integrative medicine testing. It was more specified and adjusted to ideally counter the deeper degree of illness and health dysfunction that most clients were bringing to them in practice by the late 1990s.

That brings us to the current completely updated Kelley program, as practiced by Dr. William Kelley and Pamela McDougle from the late 1990s onward. You will see there are key differences in this program compared to what is extant, practiced, and published from earlier decades because, again, *the program needed to evolve in order to keep pace with a changing world and health reality for most individuals.*

In this work, we will detail many key points and elements of the program so that it can, more or less, be followed and completed at home by individuals who need help (preferably aided by a versed clinician), who perhaps have decided to augment conventional care OR forgo conventional therapies, who have been told they have no other additional conventional options available to them, and/or who are perhaps continuing "alternative" cancer care support primarily at home that they first began at an "outside of the box" clinic. It also serves as a detailed reference guide for clinicians looking to implement the program in their practice to help individuals. We will also touch on the scientific underpinnings of the original work and connect it to where it has gone today so a continuity of evolution is clear and logical for the reader.

*NOTE: This book is NOT meant to be a critique of the current "cancer care model," other "alternative cancer therapies," or even a critique of Kelley's original work.*

This is, first and foremost, a care resource for those in great need to utilize, reference, and inform themselves (or someone they know) on how to work on their health and underlying patterns of physiological dysfunction common in cancer diagnoses.

One thing to keep in mind when working with cancer patients, or if you yourself have cancer: remember that a cancer case is "never just cancer." Typically, it has taken many months, if not years, of tumor development before the tumor has become large enough to be found with conventional imaging, testing, etc. *In this time, emotional traumas, digestive issues, nutritional deficits and imbalances, hormonal imbalances, poor lifestyle habits, inadequate sleep, infections, dental problems, toxicity issues, and more have often been mounting, thereby undermining one's health and allowing the body to break down into decay, disease, and chronic imbalance, resulting in that dreaded six-letter word: CANCER.*

For those of you that have familiarity with the field of homeopathy, which is more than 200 years old, the cancer "miasm" is a circumstantial, all-encompassing state a person moves into as their health gradually breaks down. This is typically preceded by several other miasms that each feature their own constellation of various health issues and associated symptoms and illnesses. These miasmatic conditions can have strong tendencies through family lines, which sometimes can partly explain why certain "conditions" may "run in families," as we often talk about in Western medicine.

If these earlier miasmatic states (such as "Psoric") are not corrected and/or are simply suppressed via typical allopathic suppressive medications (which is how we typically "treat" in conventional medicine—i.e., take this pill for this symptom, etc.), ultimately we continue to move to a place of greater decay and dysfunction (as the root causes of these issues were not truly addressed and balanced through nutritional and lifestyle interventions, etc.) until arriving at this highly dysfunctional and self-destructive cancer miasmal state. The father of homeopathy, Dr. Samuel Hahnemann, predicted this telling disease constellation sequence over 200 years ago, yet conventional medicine has yet to really pay attention to or take seriously this enormously insightful body of knowledge.[1]

We almost always get earlier warning signs and preced-

___

1    https://www.medicalnewstoday.com/articles/288916; https://www.cancer.org/cancer/cancer-basics/lifetime-probability-of-developing- or-dying-from-cancer.html

ing issues to the development of cancer if we simply pay attention and look more deeply. Too often, nowadays, few people truly understand what it takes to be healthy or to regain health, and with an overly busy, distracted, and confused population in general, more than 40% of Americans can expect to receive a cancer diagnosis in their lifetime.[2] Remember, one hundred years ago, cancer was not one of the top five causes of death in the US, whereas now, it is narrowly behind heart disease as number two.[3]

So, what's changed? Well, a lot, of course. But part of the solution, in addition to becoming much more knowledgeable about health, *is also about shifting one's priorities to practicing a health-promoting lifestyle.* Most individuals are unknowingly sabotaging their own health because of a lack of knowledge, reliance on a disease-care model system of health care (versus one that is truly about "health care"), and lastly, a lack of prioritization of one's health.

The Complete Updated Kelley Protocol is a toolset to help just that: to help one work on regaining true, vibrant health so that disease will not want to or be able to flourish. It should be noted this is a self-empowerment process and a journey that will take some time. Remember, it likely took YEARS for your health to break down to the point of you getting a cancer diagnosis; it will take a number of months to

---

2   https://www.cdc.gov/nchs/data/dvs/lead1900_98.pdf; https://www.livescience.com/21213-leading-causes-of-death-in-the-u-s-since-1900-infographic.html

3   https://www.cdc.gov/nchs/data/dvs/lead1900_98.pdf; https://www.livescience.com/21213-leading-causes-of-death-in-the-u-s-since-1900-infographic.html

several years for you to be able to hopefully regain it. Subsequently, patience and persistence are key in this process.

**Lastly, remember your body always wants to heal and self-correct, whether you are 30 years old or 90 years old!** We just have to know enough to help it, apply it, and then *give it some time to do what it inherently knows to do.* One of the key tenets of naturopathic medicine notes this: *Vis Medicatrix Naturae.* This translates to "The Healing Power of Nature"—trusting in the body's inherent wisdom to heal itself.

We hope this work is able to help many achieve just that: to help them take back their health and their quality of life through this deep-acting, comprehensive, at-home health promotion program. We are excited to share this knowledge and gift that Dr. Kelley gave back to the world for the benefit of many who may have little to no other options in their medical time of need.

**Dr. Eric Wood, ND, MA and Pamela McDougle, NC**

# About the Authors

**Pamela McDougle, NC** (nutritional consultant), was Dr. William Kelley's last student to train and work with him in practice in the 1990s. She brings 30+ years of clinical experience as a clinical nutritionist practitioner working with the Kelley program in thousands of diverse cases across North America and beyond. Pamela began her nutritional training in 1990 under the health pioneer Dr. Ann Wigmore at the Hippocrates Health Institute in Boston, Massachusetts. She later studied at the Life Science Institute. During the last three decades, she has accumulated a wealth of experience and expertise in nutrition, digestive health, and cancer especially, and has partnered with other notable clinicians and practices across North America and Europe in bringing the knowledge of the Kelley program to practitioners near and far.

**Dr. Eric Wood, ND, MA,** is an Associate Professor of Integrative and Functional medicine at John Patrick University and Adjunct Faculty in Naturopathic Medicine at National University of Healthcare Sciences and Holistic Nutrition at the American College of Healthcare Sciences. He is a practicing naturopathic doctor licensed in Washington, DC & Minnesota, with more than fifteen years of experience in practice and the natural/integrative health industry. He has worked with some of the leading supplement and natural medicine organizations in the country and beyond, including Life Extension as an integrative cancer specialist, Neuroscience Inc., Physician's Choice, Primal Labs, Ben's Natural Health, and more. A published author, musician, and accomplished speaker with guest appearances on various webinars, podcasts, and national networks, including ABC, NBC, Fox, The CW, and other stations, he was also featured in an international documentary titled "Food, Health, and You." A graduate of the Canadian College of Naturopathic Medicine, he completed a year-long fellowship in environmental medicine via Environmental Medicine Education International (i.e., EMEI Global) in 2022 and has received additional training at Harvard's Benson Henry Institute for Mind-Body Medicine and Georgetown's Food as Medicine program. Dr. Wood was Pamela McDougle's last student trained in the Kelley program and has been working with clients across North America and beyond since completing his training with her in 2015.

# CHAPTER ONE

## Medical History: Where We've Come From Theoretically and Politically, and Where We've Arguably Gone Wrong

As a professor, I have lectured on diverse medical topics, but one of the common threads I focus on is giving people a deep understanding of where we are today by looking back at medical history. A key concept that arises when we look back in time and explains so much of where we are today is that of "terrain theory" versus "germ theory." This is one that I frequently come back to again and again, and refers to a schism that happened within the practicing medical field relatively recently (and by recent, for the sake of conversation, I'm going to say the last 150 years). If we understand this schism, so much of what is still going on, good and bad, makes so much more sense. It also explains why we need to continue to evolve the medical and health paradigms because, in some ways, we are still very penned in by and heavily influenced by monumental medical theories and accompanying political/

industry agendas that have happened during this timeframe.

A lot of what has transpired medically in much of the West over the last one hundred years plus can be linked back, on some level, to this fracture in medical theory and practice, which involved the notable Louis Pasteur and medical contemporaries such as Antoine Beauchamp. Without getting too heavily mired in medical history, many of you may know Louis Pasteur (and Robert Koch) as the "fathers of modern germ theory" (i.e., understanding that microbes can cause disease and illness). This theory suggests that most disease is caused by microbes (i.e., bacteria and viruses), and if we eradicate/destroy these microbes, the associated diseases will disappear and health will return. Eventually, this perspective became largely adopted by mainstream Western medicine in the late 1800s, first in Europe and quickly after in North America, and allowed for the burgeoning modern pharmaceutical industry to become so centralized and codified in the practice of medicine, initially with the introduction of antibiotics.

Remember, at this time, pharmaceutical-based interventions in medicine were not the norm. Rather, herbal medicine, homeopathy, hydrotherapy, and other "natural medicine approaches" were common, first-line therapies that many individuals sought and practiced across North America.[4] In the first two decades of the twentieth century, there were dozens of naturopathic and homeopathic medical schools across the US training practitioners in natural

---

4    Murray, Michael and Joseph Pizzorno. *Encyclopedia of Natural Medicine*. Prima Publishing, 1998.

therapies/approaches.[5] This was before the rise of Big Pharma and financially/politically influential reports such as the Flexnor Report (from Johns Hopkins University) came out, dramatically changing the medical education and practice landscape across North America for many decades to follow. These movements also effectively wiped out the majority of these schools and practitioners for a good half-century.[6]

"Germ theory" stood in stark contrast to another theory, "terrain theory," of which many other esteemed colleagues of Pasteur's (such as fellow French Academy of Sciences member Antoine Beauchamp) were much bigger proponents. In sum, the idea of "terrain theory" suggests that the state of the health of an individual (which is notably heavily influenced by and "built" on good nutrition, adequate rest, good structural alignment, clean living [i.e., lack of toxins/poisons], good emotional health, etc.) is highly influential in protecting against pathogens taking root and allowing the body to break down to the point where they become entrenched and disease-promoting. Notably, "terrain theory" medical practice is very similar to how many modern holistic providers today (such as naturopaths, chiropractors, functional medicine or "holistic" medical doctors, nutritionists, and acupuncturists) view health and treat patients.

Had terrain theory instead of germ theory become so central to the practice of "modern medicine" in the late 1800s,

---

5    Murray, Michael and Joseph Pizzorno. *Encyclopedia of Natural Medicine*. Prima Publishing, 1998.

6    Campion, F. "AMA and U.S. Health Policy Since 1940." *JAMA Publications*, 1984; https://www.ncbi.nlm.nih.gov/pmc/articles/ PMC3543812/.

we might be looking at a *VERY* different medical landscape across much of the world today—one where nutrition, detoxification, exercise therapy, emotional healing, and more were instead the first-line cornerstones that we went to in order to help individuals recover from a diverse number of situations and ailments even with "traditional medical providers."

However, across the West, this isn't our reality, at least yet, and we see germ-theory-derived medical practices and perspectives, to varying degrees, dominating Western countries' modern medical systems.[7] That said, many shifts in the health care landscape have been happening in the last forty years with the return of more and more natural, now scientifically validated therapies and the boom of "alternative/complementary" medicine. In this timeframe, more and more holistic and integrative health care programs, schools, and practitioners have become available to the public.

This has been driven by the demand of more and more individuals recognizing the considerable shortcomings of modern-day, traditional medical practice, with its overreliance on germ theory-derived, reductionistic practices. The rise of the internet over the last 30 years has only accelerated individuals' ability to find and seek out such care as well.

And indeed, this is probably why you're reading this book: because you're looking for other options that you're not

---

7   That said, due to a variety of reasons such as post-WWII constitutional reforms, some countries such as Germany, Switzerland, and France have integrated more use of herbal medicines, homeopathy, and nutrition into their standard medical care versus countries such as the US, Canada, Australia, and others.

going to get offered through your traditional providers, and you know, on some level, that your nutritional status, your toxicity levels, your emotional health, and more REALLY DO MATTER when it pertains to your health and overcoming illness!

Ultimately, as committed practitioners to patient well-being, we want to have as many sound, scientifically rational interventions and therapies from ALL parts of medicine accessible to potentially use for individuals in need, and to not get bogged down by ideological and political schisms in medicine. But for too long, valuable, powerful, and deeply healing natural medicines and therapies have often been castigated and relegated to the fringes of medicine due to lack of proper consideration, impediments to funding well-designed research studies, lack of understanding by those in positions of power and influence, and more. It's time these options also have their proper place, front and center, to help those in deep need of health restoration, along with the best parts of allopathic medicine as well.

It is truly time we embrace all the "tools" in our medical "toolbox" from **all parts of medicine**, whether as a patient or a provider alike, whether allopathic, naturopathic, or whatnot, for the future good of medicine, to ultimately best serve our patients and ourselves. We **cannot** wait for politics and legislation to catch up, which are reactive at best and often take decades, if not generations, to catch up to where extant research is.[8]

---

8    https://www.ncbi.nlm.nih.gov/pmc/articles/PMC3241518/

# CHAPTER TWO

## The Underpinnings of the Metabolic Theory of Cancer, Rethinking Immunity, and Pancreatic Enzymes' Roles in Cancer

For many decades, the assumed theory surrounding cancer has been one focused on DNA damage as being the centerpiece of "what goes wrong in a cell" and how cancer can develop from a highly damaged cell. This is also the theory around which many conventional cancer therapies have developed—to namely destroy these aberrant, highly mutated cells. However, in recent decades, this theory has been increasingly challenged by what we term the "metabolic theory" of cancer, which stems back multiple generations to early, groundbreaking researchers like Otto Warburg.

Instead of focusing on DNA damage as the centerpiece to understanding the genesis of cancer's development and uncontrollable spread, the metabolic theory instead posits that this is really a mitochondrial damage issue. In this case, a cell's mitochondria have become so damaged that they're no longer able to effectively use oxygen as a fuel generator (to produce cellular energy called "ATP" or adenosine triphosphate), and hence, they revert to a more primitive and much less efficient form of energy creation (driven by fermenting primarily carbohydrates) to produce ATP termed "anaerobic metabolism." Notably, mitochondrial DNA is far LESS protected than nuclear DNA, as nuclear DNA is protected via a considerable cellular wall that surrounds it, whereas mitochondrial DNA is only shielded via the thin cell membrane that separates the mitochondria from the rest of the cell and its respective organelles.

While the focus of this book is NOT to debate the myriad of points related to this *significant* potential paradigm shift on how we think about cancer, if we think about things that do damage to both mitochondria and nuclear DNA, how we mitigate that and overcome it, we come back to similar strategies: increased antioxidant intake, reduction of toxin load and exposure, reduction in the generation of free radical species created by way of many stressors, increased good nutrient consumption, and optimizing cellular repair strategies through proper rest, stress management, reduction of damaging environmental forces, possibly IV therapies, and more. This is, essentially, "terrain theory" work!

Concurrently, it has also been presupposed that the primary immune system fixture of the body in eradicating cancer cells are natural killer cells, a key type of potent white blood cell. And indeed, while these are powerful immune cells capable of destroying a variety of cancer cells, viruses, and bacteria, Dr. Kelley believed, like other prominent researchers before him, such as John Beard, that pancreatic enzymes were also a prominent player in the defense system of the body in protecting against cancer cells growing out of hand. Since then, research has gradually mounted supporting this theory and a number of prominent scientists and medical professionals over the generations have concurred, including Dr. Francis Pottenger, Dr. Franklin Shivley, Dr. Linda Isaacs, Dr. Nicholas Gonzalez, Dr. Lloyd Old, former director of the Sloan Kettering Memorial Cancer Research Institute, and more recently, Dr. George Yu, MD, from whom we have included a medical opinion paper link in the below footnote, describing his experience with enzymes, cancer, and more.[9, 10] He lends some informed hypotheses as to why we continue to see benefits from protease enzyme therapy in this paper, and we've included several of his diagrams where he references illustrating potential mechanisms of action. As with the majority of 'alternative' and 'complementary' therapies, the drive is to get more high-quality research completed to elucidate more exact mechanisms of action of benefit, as the late Dr Gonzalez attempted to do when practicing.

To begin, it's helpful to do a little review, especially for those without a considerable medical background. Enzymes are primarily produced by our pancreas to help continue digesting food in the small intestine that has first been received by the stomach, where the first phases of breaking apart proteins and sanitizing our food occur.

---

9    http://www.enzyme-facts.com/enzymes-history; https://www.researchgate.net/publication/5863901_Cancer_is_a_somatic_cell_pregnancy ; Beard, J: "The Enzyme Treatment of Cancer" London: Chatto and Windus, 1911.

10   https://yufoundation.org/the-systemic-of-protease-enzyme-in-cancer

Different enzymes that our body produces will work on digesting fats (i.e., lipases), carbs (i.e., amylase, cellulase, lactase, etc.), or proteins (i.e., trypsin, chymotrypsin, pepsin, etc.), and by action of these enzymes, these 'macronutrients' from your food are broken into smaller and smaller pieces in your small intestine. This is so they are ultimately the right size for absorption into the blood/body via finger-like projections along your intestines' wall, called 'villi.' Many people nowadays have become familiar with enzymes in that they can help with routine indigestion after eating. Well, enzymes indeed do that but can also be powerfully influential in diminishing pain and inflammation, and, as discussed below, in facilitating what we term 'autophagy' (i.e., breakdown of unwanted metabolic tissue/debris).[11]

The enzymes being injected into the small intestine via a duct from the pancreas can *also be absorbed through the walls of the intestines* where they can travel to other parts of the body, helping to break down fibrous scar tissue from injury, and as Beard and others suggest, cancer cells. These enzymes, by traveling via the bloodstream, can arrive at the site of the tumor and work on digesting the specific proteins of the tumor mass without harming the body's own healthy tissues due to believed differences in the orientation of proteins within tumor cells (i.e., 'right-handed' orientation) vs. healthy cells (i.e., 'left-handed' orientation). John Beard noted this more

---

11  The German company and brand Wobenzym has been undertaking and reviewing research on enzymes' ability to help with pain, inflammation, and other complaints for nearly sixty years, notably. See: https://www.wobenzym.de/ for more details and research.

than one hundred years ago in his work![12] This allows the enzymes, over time, to gradually 'liquefy' the tumor(s) and make them more visible to the body's immune system for concurrent destruction. Ultimately, this metabolic debris is gradually broken down and excreted out of the body through the various routes of filtering and excretion (i.e., namely, filtering by the liver and kidneys to be excreted out via the bowels).

## What a Discovery by Beard!

Given this perspective and belief of Beard, Kelley, and others before him, it would stand to reason that supplementing with pancreatic enzymes (notably at considerable dosages) could act in a beneficial fashion to boost immunosurveillance and eradication of tumor cells, as references noted earlier in footnote nine and this section suggest. This is exactly why pancreatic enzymes became a cornerstone in this protocol: they offer a substantial boon to helping the body fight off cancer cells.

Dr. Yu has developed and referenced several useful diagrams and studies to illustrate how and where we believe enzymes play a vital role as an essential piece of a comprehensive approach in fighting cancer. See next page:

---

12  Beard, John. "The Enzyme Treatment of Cancer and Its Scientific Basis." London, 1911.

## Multi-modalities of Cancer Suppression & Kill

George Yu, M.D.

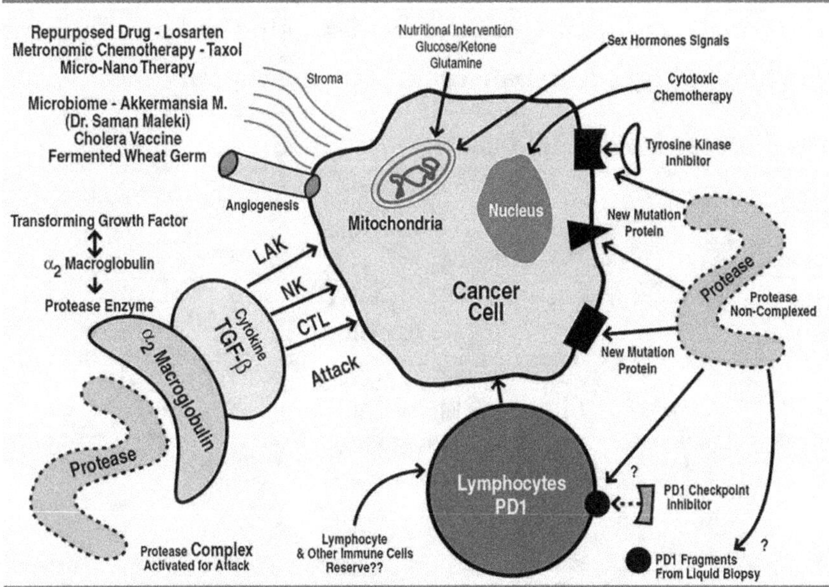




Harthun, N.L. Slingluff, C.L., J of Immunotherapy 21 (2) 85-94,1998
199   Leipner J.. Saller Reinhard. Systemic Enzyme in Oncology. Drugs 2000 April 59(4)769-780


The key here is that they may play an especially vital role in combatting new protein mutations in cancer cell antigens, making old therapies less effective and making it harder for the immune system to 'read' the antigens and recognize the cells as cancer and subsequently target them for destruction. Please see the referenced papers in the following footnote about the relationship between protease enzymes and alpha 2 macroglobulin, and note the following about what we already know about alpha 2 macroglobulin: it is mainly produced by the liver and is locally synthesized by macrophages, fibroblasts, and adrenocortical cells. It is an antiprotease and is able to inactivate an enormous variety of proteinases while additionally functioning as an inhibitor of fibrinolysis by inhibiting plasmin and kallikrein.[13] Understanding this lends us additional insight into the proposed benefits and mechanisms of action of high-dose pancreatic enzyme therapy.

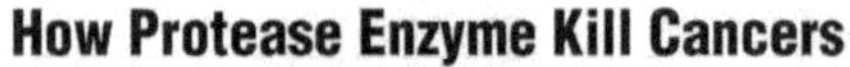

### How Protease Enzyme Kill Cancers

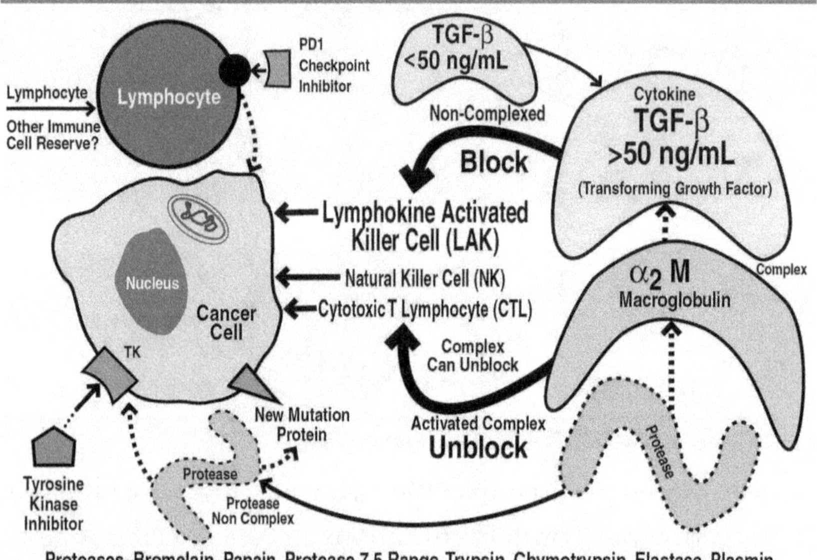




200    Harthun, N.L. Slingluff, C.L., J of Immunotherapy 21 (2) 85-94,1998
     Leipner J., Saller Reinhard, Systemic Enzyme In Onocology, Drugs 2000 April 59(4)769-780


Furthermore, Dr. Yu notes: "The key is that these powerful protease enzymes can cross the intestinal blood barrier and are not harmful to the host body but seem to have an indiscriminate ability to digest or denature foreign proteins as I have witnessed in my postoperative surgical experience with dead and residual protein and blood fragments as a 'Paceman' effect on wounds and ecchymoses."

In fact, Kelley went further in explaining why enzyme therapy is so important for many cancer patients: due to im-

---

13   https://pubmed.ncbi.nlm.nih.gov/34970276; https://www.ncbi.nlm.nih.gov/pmc/articles/PMC8897276; https://www.ncbi.nlm.nih.gov/pmc/articles/PMC6679887/

balances in how they were living, they had disturbed the autonomic nervous system balance and subsequent functioning of the body, typically resulting in inefficient digestion and decreased pancreatic function. Subsequently, this resulted in diminishing production of said enzymes that were absorbed into the bloodstream by way of the GI tract, especially when there were not substantial amounts of food present (which would utilize many of these enzymes to help facilitate its breakdown), leading to a greater opportunity for cancer cells to escape this important defensive system.

## What a Profound Theory Indeed

Given today's rampant abundance of digestive and gastrointestinal problems, prediabetes, and diabetes (whereby the pancreas is considerably underfunctioning), it would only stand that for many, their levels of pancreatic enzymes available to function in this important 'immunosurveillance fashion' would be suboptimal, thus making them potentially more susceptible to cancer cells being able to escape eradication and to proliferate. Incidentally, in practice, I have observed a high concordance of chronic gastrointestinal/digestive problems proceeding the diagnosis of a variety of cancers in hundreds of clients over the years. Given all of this, *it would seem that our lifestyles, digestive health, and dietary practices are considerably fueling this cancer epidemic and certainly should be taken much more seriously for both prevention AS WELL as part of treatment* for those needing cancer care. Dr Kelley certainly believed so.

## A Note on European Enzyme Research

Of the limited published literature we have involving enzyme therapy studied clinically in a clinic or hospital setting, the overwhelming majority comes from the German-speaking countries of Europe. An excellent review article published by the University of Zurich, Switzerland, more than twenty years ago chronicled a number of smaller studies using varying strengths and types of pancreatic enzymes to further elucidate what we might expect from targeted pancreatic enzyme therapy.[14] The review article noted a number of prospective benefits with the use of enzyme therapy, including concurrent administration of chemotherapy and/or radiation regimens. Some examples include: fewer side effects with and better tolerance of such therapies was observed in multiple studies; improvements in liver enzyme levels, as well as t lymphocyte counts; fewer metastases; and, to varying degrees, improvements in life expectancy and more individuals living beyond 42 months.

As mentioned before, more well-designed clinical trials are needed to further elucidate expectations, more understanding of mechanisms of action, and whatnot. But the studies we have, the understanding of the immune system and cancer cell physiology, as well as the chronicled anecdotal work of Dr. Kelley and his students, all point to the observation that there really is something potent and important about enzymes as an ally in the fight against cancer AND that these can be used in conjunction with conventional therapies.

---

14　Drugs: 2000, April. "Systemic Enzyme Therapy in Oncology": 769-780.

# CHAPTER THREE

## The Old Program and Why It Needed to Change Along with Our Changing and Sickening World

As we alluded to earlier on, this program has evolved over the years because it had to. What worked in the 1960s and 70s for many people simply wasn't working as well by the 1990s. I fear this will need to happen again as, sadly, most people continue to get sicker and sicker on average, as so many of us working with clients are seeing. As discussed, this is primarily due to negative changes in many individuals' habits and exposures over subsequent decades—from the consumption of more processed foods and refined sugars to increasing levels and varied routes of environmental toxicants, declining amounts and quality of sleep since the 1960s, and more chronic stressors. Thus, the need for revamping and reconsidering certain elements of the program came to be out of necessity to do better for clients.

So, you might ask, are things really that different dietarily and lifestyle habit-wise now versus the 1960s/'70s (or even earlier)? Well, aside from obvious changes that we're all aware of, such as the types and greater usage of personal technology (laptops, cell phones, tablets, etc.), all of which were nonexistent in the '60s and '70s, and each produces electromagnetic frequency (EMF) radiation, different fashions, different cars, etc., **there are many PROFOUND changes that have occurred related to lifestyle and dietary habits, sleep, toxin exposure, and stressors**. A considerable portion of this chapter will be devoted to illustrating this and connecting why we need to do better on so many of these fronts for our health's sake, because, sadly, most of them are going in the wrong direction.

But as with any change process, the first step in changing things is to first gain awareness that there is even a problem. And that's the tricky thing about these changes: when they have happened incrementally over the years, they're a lot harder to notice and pinpoint, and thus, the "obviousness" of them becomes obscured.

So that's where I'm going to start: by namely reviewing and highlighting some of these shifts in these important areas and connecting the dots as to why these changes are significant to our health, how they have potentially impacted the program, and what you can do to minimize some of these negative shifts in your own life and your family's lives, whether or not you are doing "the Kelley program" or working with a patient in such a situation. To better illustrate some of these shifts in the last fifty years, I'm going to review some of the major areas in habits and exposures where we're seeing disturbing and/or negative changes that have the potential to markedly influence health by detailing some data and graphics. As appropriate, I will also connect these points to the protocol and how they may have impacted changes in the protocol over time.

## Nutritional Shifts

One of the most profound shifts that's happened in the food landscape over the last several generations is the large-scale introduction of genetically modified organisms (GMOs) in 1997. Another concurrent big shift has been a more gradual shift away from cooking in the home and "making things from scratch" (or near scratch) to eating out more and eating more processed, heavily refined, and often sugar-laden foods. The following graphics chart both the introduction of GMOs, the concordance of increased health issues, and also the frequency of individuals eating out on a weekly basis in the US.

## The Correlation of the Introduction of GMOs, Roundup Pesticide, and a Number of Health Issues' Incidences[15]

It's hard to explain the exponentially marked increase in various illnesses as "coincidental" when you look at the data over the last twenty-five-plus years since GMO foods and Roundup were widely introduced in the 1990s. It is really quite striking and frankly scary, to say the least. Below are just a FEW of the many publicly available graphics of the plot points between various illnesses and the types and amounts of GMOs introduced since the mid-1990s.[16]

---

15  http://www.organic-systems.org/journal/92/JOS_Volume-9_Number-2_Nov_2014-Swanson-et-al.pdf

16  http://www.organic-systems.org/journal/92/JOS_Volume-9_Number-2_Nov_2014-Swanson-et-al.pdf

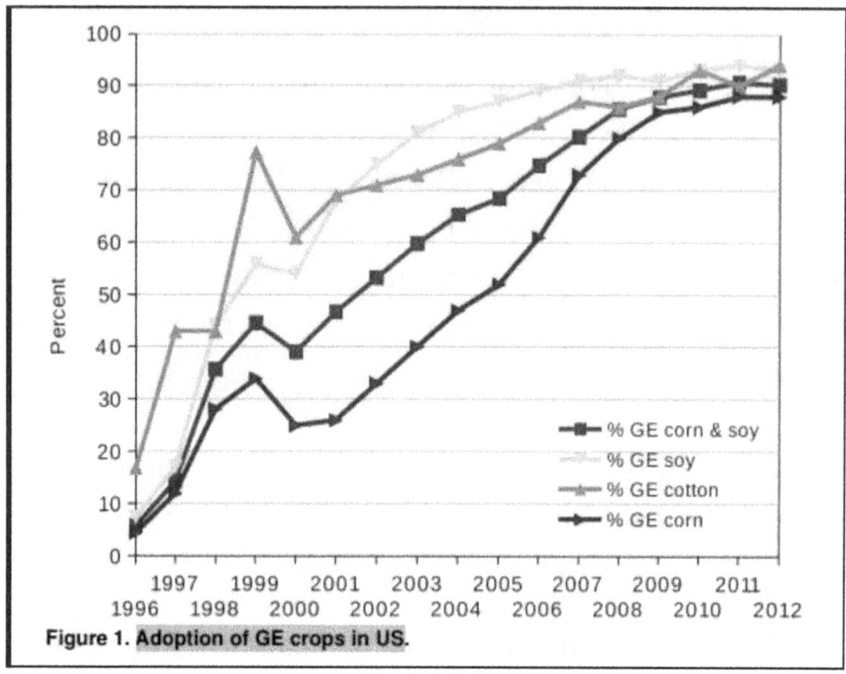



**Figure 1. Adoption of GE crops in US.**

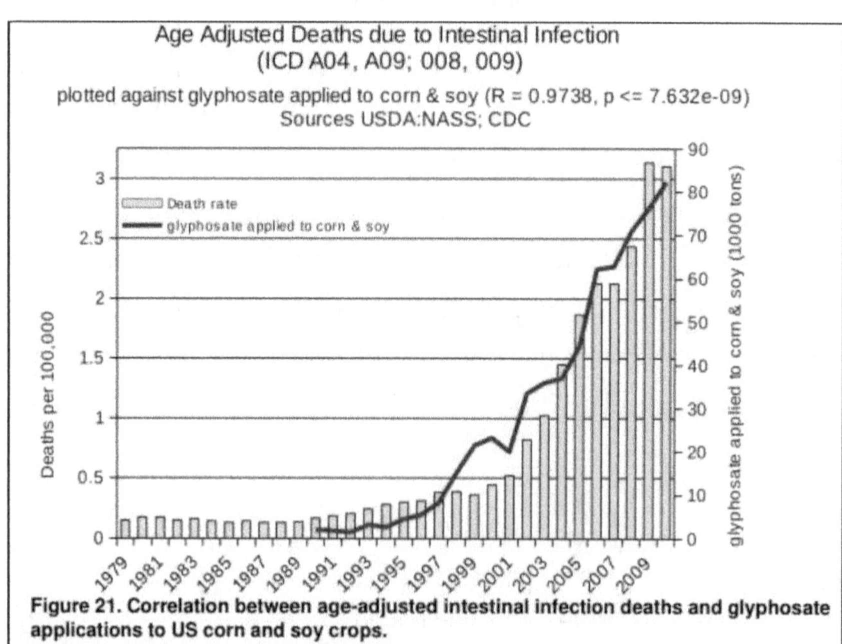



**Figure 21. Correlation between age-adjusted intestinal infection deaths and glyphosate applications to US corn and soy crops.**

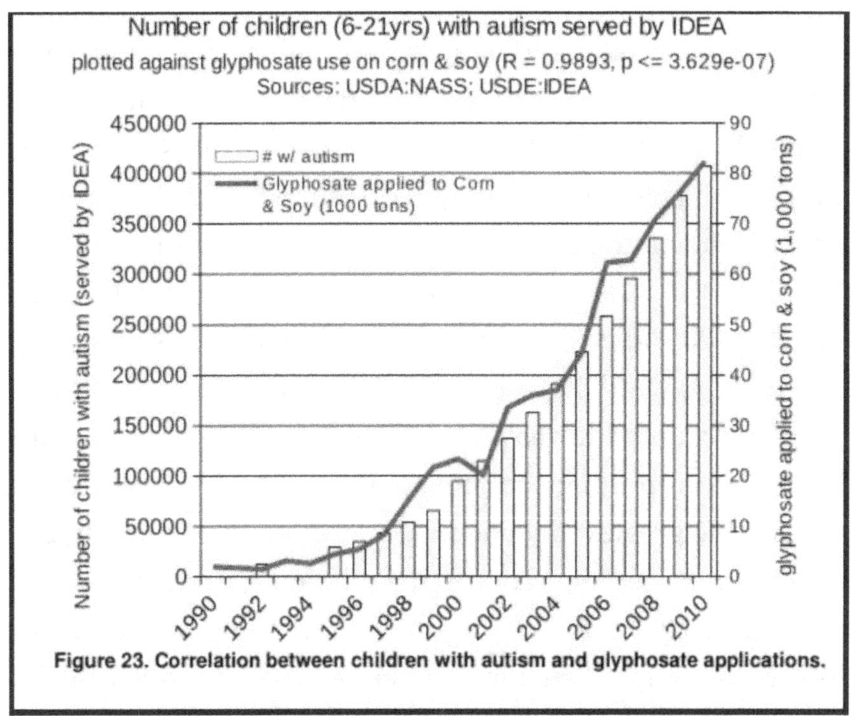



**Figure 23. Correlation between children with autism and glyphosate applications.**

When you think about it, is it really surprising, given that Roundup is meant to KILL small pests by specifically rupturing the lumen of their bellies, that this could hurt and negatively impact people, specifically impacting gut health, immunity, and immune regulation (especially given that the bulk of the immune system lies within the intestinal tract)?

Given the omnipresence of GMOs and pesticides now in use in conventional food, the Kelley program insists on all organic, minimally and/or nonprocessed foods that are also non-irradiated, as we cannot be damaging ourselves when we are trying to heal concurrently by a compromised food supply!

## The Frequency of Eating Out Over Time, 1889 until 2009[17]

When we take a look at dietary habits over more than a century, it is so easy to see how dramatically things have changed societally. More recent research illustrates that the percentage of daily energy consumed from home food sources and time spent in food preparation decreased significantly for all socioeconomic groups between 1965–1966 and 2007–2008 ($p \leq 0.001$), with the largest declines occurring between 1965 and 1992. In 2007–2008, foods from the home supply accounted for 65% to 72% of total daily energy, with 54% to 57% reporting cooking activities. Low-income groups showed the greatest decline in the proportion of cooking but consumed more daily energy from home sources and spent more time cooking than high-income individuals in 2007–2008 ($p \leq 0.001$).[18] You can see below just how much things have changed since, especially in the early 1960s when fast food consumption was still a minimal percentage of the diet.

---

17  Thankfully, it appears the trend of Americans eating more takeout and restaurant food has leveled off and is little changed since 2008. See: https://news.gallup.com/poll/201710/americans-dining-frequency-little-changed-2008.aspx

18  https://www.ncbi.nlm.nih.gov/pmc/articles/PMC3639863/

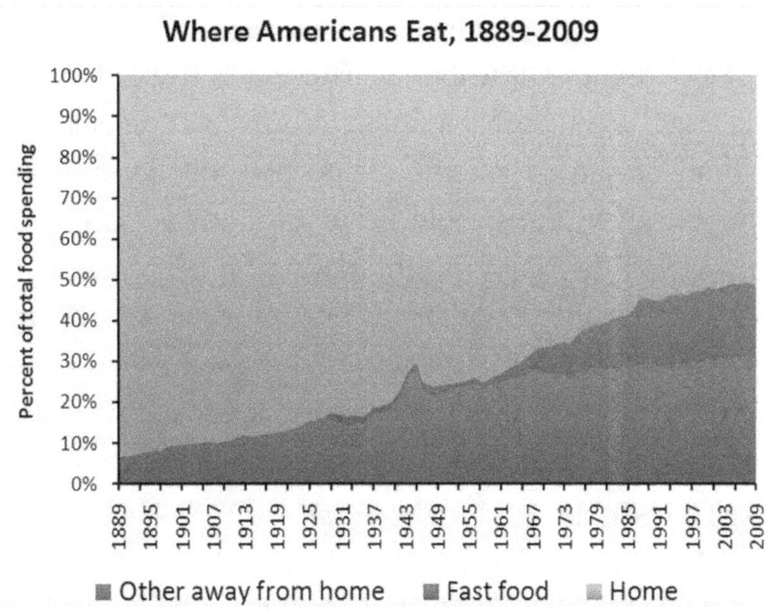


The data referenced in the graph above comes from USDA figures; notably, fast-food expenditures were not tracked before 1929. A few trends of note emerge here:

I. Ninety-three percent of food was consumed at home in 1889, and most of that was homemade from scratch.

II. In 2009, barely half (51%) of food was consumed at home; the rest was consumed in either full-service or fast-food restaurants. It's likely that a high proportion of what was consumed at home was processed food.

III. Fast food was not a significant household expenditure before 1960, after which it rapidly gained in popularity. Today, fast food accounts for 18% of total food expenditures.

The obesity epidemic began between 1970 and 1980, at the same time that fast food consumption began to majorly spike and has continued since.[19] Of course, eating out doesn't inherently mean people are eating poor-quality junk food. However, given the sizable percentage of fast-food restaurants, as well as less than optimally prepared and sourced foods used in the majority of restaurants, it is intrinsically very difficult in most parts of the country to eat close to ideally when you go out to the majority of restaurants. Here in South Florida, which is a fairly health-conscious locale compared to many parts of the country in my experience, I still have a rather short list of restaurants I would recommend or eat at if one is trying to eat truly "healthy."

Thus, given how frequently food is negatively compromised when prepared commercially, those individuals on the Kelley program will largely be eating homemade foods or minimally supplementing their diet with extremely high-quality, commercially available foodstuffs that follow the very particular dietary guidelines of the program, which will be detailed in a later chapter. This may be quite an adjustment for some people when you consider the food consumption patterns of recent years, but nonetheless, if we all once ate this way, it certainly is possible again, especially if your health may depend on it!

---

19   https://wholehealthsource.blogspot.com/2011/05/fast-food-weight-gain-and-insulin.html; https://www.healthline.com/nutrition/11-graphs-that-show-what-is-wrong-with-modern-diet#section9

## Comparing Sugar Consumption over the Last 300 Years in Correlation with Obesity Prevalence

As the saying goes, a picture is worth a thousand words, and wow, does this graphic illustrate a disturbing trend, to say the least. Consumption of refined, nutrient-poor carbohydrates has been on the rise for most of the last 300 years plus, and with that, obesity has skyrocketed, especially in the latter of the twentieth century, now into the twenty-first.

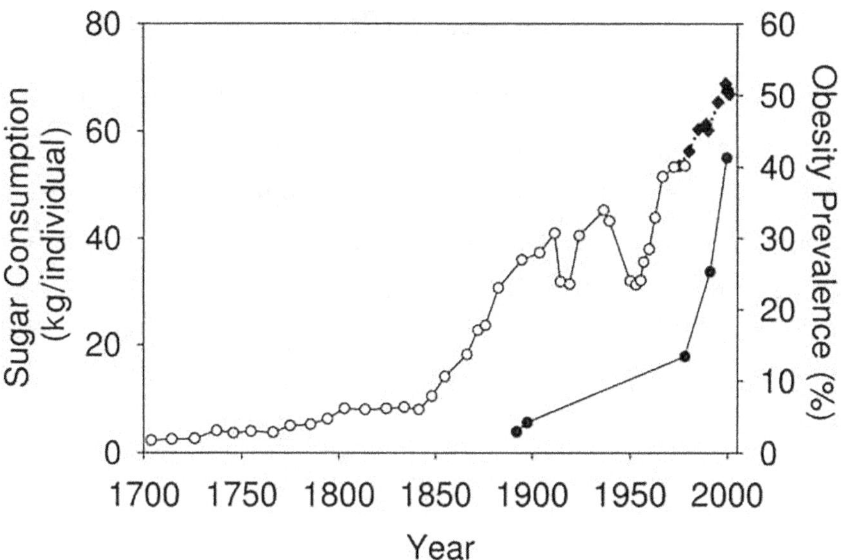


**Source:** Johnson, R.J., et al. "Potential role of sugar (fructose) in the epidemic of hypertension, obesity and the metabolic syndrome, diabetes, kidney disease, and cardiovascular disease." *The American Journal of Clinical Nutrition,* 86, no. 4 (2007): 899-906.

We know that processed sugar and refined carbohydrates, in general, wreak havoc on the function and durability of our pancreas organ, which is chiefly responsible for helping us regulate blood sugar AND, remember, is responsible for producing those all too important pancreatic enzymes. Is it any wonder that the incidence of type II diabetes has concurrently paralleled the rise in obesity during this time? I think not.

Thus, it should come as no surprise that refined carbohydrates and especially refined sugars are completely omitted in the Kelley program.

## Overall Health Status and Marked Changes in Chronic Illness over Time

Never in recent generations has health decline begun so early or so sharply, as recent research suggests. The graphic below shows an alarming trend that by age 27, a pronounced downward swing has already begun in health matrices, according to research conducted on millennials (born between 1981–1996).[20]

---

20  https://www.dailymail.co.uk/health/article-6981315/Millennials-health-plummets-age-27-study-finds.html

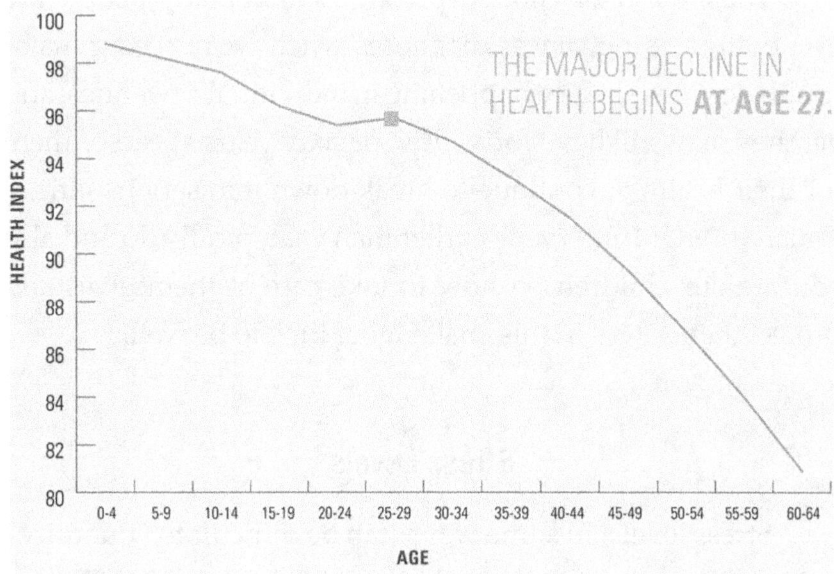


These various indices of health decline are many when we look closely at the data—from rising rates of infertility, diabetes, obesity, cancer, heart disease, headaches, fatigue, and much, much more.

It's scary to think what this early decline means for adults attempting to have and raise children at later and later ages, taking care of aging parents, and sustaining careers. At some point, things are going to break…and it's happening earlier and earlier. We have been witnessing more and more cases of serious illness, including cancer, in clients in their forties, thirties, and even late twenties in recent years, and not coincidentally, professional screening recommendations also have been dropping in age for illnesses such as colon cancer.[21]

---

21  https://www.uchicagomedicine.org/forefront/cancer-articles/new-guidelines-lower-colorectal-screening-age-from-50-to-45

Thus, it's really not surprising that so many people are eventually getting cancer diagnoses when we're seeing major health declines already happening in individuals' twenties, and yet they may still have forty, fifty, or sixty years ahead of them for their health to continue to break down into serious illness. Thus, we MUST intervene earlier than we typically do and also educate our children on how to take care of themselves and protect themselves in this challenging time to be well.

## Stress Levels

Stress levels, in some ways, can be difficult to "quantify" because, in part, stress is a subjective, highly contextual term. What may stress one person out at one moment in time may not bother someone else and vice versa. So what may be a more useful way to talk about this (and compare across the decades) might be to take a look at some of the more commonly recognized stressors common in many individuals' lives that have been measured and/or quantified in some ways over the years. These could include: 1) the financial costs of maintaining a middle-class lifestyle and correlating average income with inflation over the years to understanding purchasing power for various individuals of different generations (and thus how negative changes in such can add stress to working families to try and keep up with all the expense demands); 2) the average amount of refined sugars, cigarettes, and/or alcohol consumed daily; and 3) the average number of exogenous chemicals individuals may be exposed to on a daily level over time. We already reviewed earlier how sugar and refined food consumption levels have changed for the worse over time; below, you will find graphics depicting the enormous increased costs of housing, education, and health care for the average American family since the 1970s before we move into discussing the disconcerting dangers of toxins that many of us are routinely encountering.

**Note:** For those not too familiar with some helpful basic economic indicator relationships, you will see terms such as inflation and the closely related purchasing power indices referenced below. In general, these are economic concepts that help us understand the relative increase of cost of goods and services versus the average income of a respective era so we can understand how "relatively expensive" something is for a person or family in a particular era versus another time. This is important especially because we cannot just compare the sheer costs of goods and services in isolation without contextualizing them relative to income, as income has also continued to rise over time (but notably more slowly than many major expenses for middle-class families, as the below graphics illustrate). Notably, as the graphic below details, in the last two generations, the average middle-class family has seen especially large increases in relative costs of health care, education, and housing, which are typically three of the biggest expenses families incur over time. This trend is putting more and more strain and stress on working adults to "pay for it all."[22] And at some point, remember, we all have our limits and can reach our breaking points when it comes to our physical and mental health.

---

22  https://www.cnbc.com/2018/04/17/how-much-more-expensive-life-is-today-than-it-was-in-1960.html; https://www.lendingtree.com/student/millennials-have-it-worse-study/

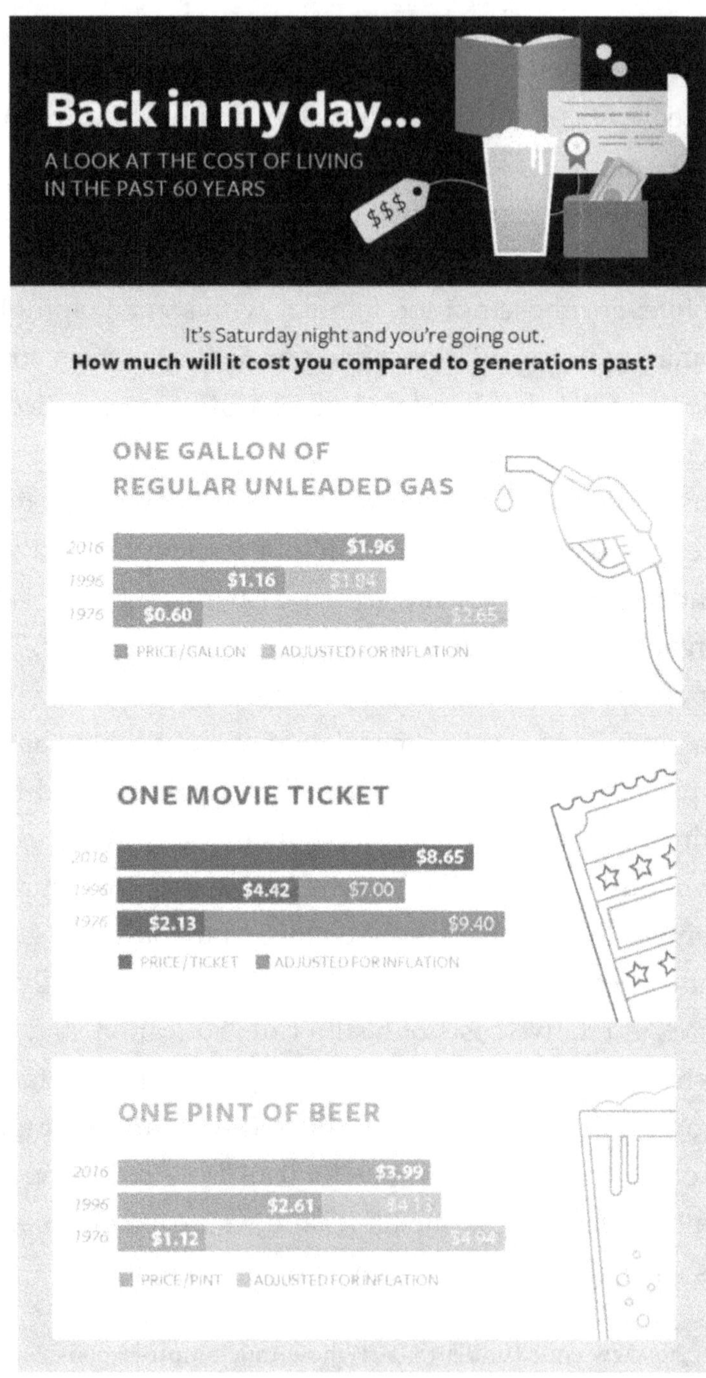
Back in my day...
A LOOK AT THE COST OF LIVING
IN THE PAST 60 YEARS
$$$
It's Saturday night and you're going out.
How much will it cost you compared to generations past?
ONE GALLON OF
REGULAR UNLEADED GAS
2016
$1.96
1996
$1.16
$1.04
1976
$0.60
$2.65
PRICE/GALLON
ADJUSTED FOR INFLATION
ONE MOVIE TICKET
2016
$8.65
1996
$4.42
$7.00
1976
$2.13
$9.40
PRICE/TICKET
ADJUSTED FOR INFLATION
ONE PINT OF BEER
2016
$3.99
1996
$2.61
$4.18
1976
$1.12
$4.94
PRICE/PINT
ADJUSTED FOR INFLATION

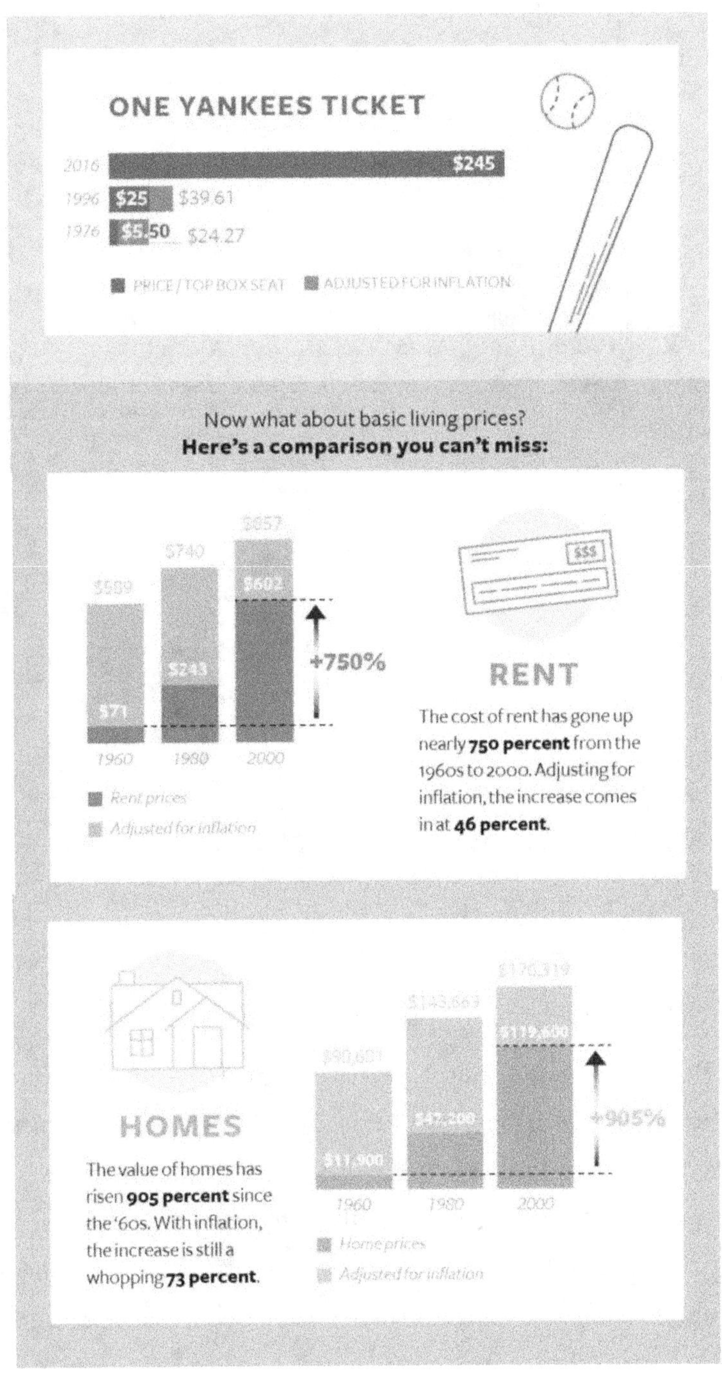
ONE YANKEES TICKET
2016
$245
1996
$25
$39.61
1976
$5.50
$24.27
PRICE/TOP BOX SEAT
ADJUSTED FOR INFLATION
Now what about basic living prices?
Here's a comparison you can't miss:
$740
$602
$243
$71
1960
1980
2000
+750%
Rent prices
Adjusted for inflation
RENT
The cost of rent has gone up nearly 750 percent from the 1960s to 2000. Adjusting for inflation, the increase comes in at 46 percent.
$119,600
$11,900
1960
1980
2000
+905%
HOMES
The value of homes has risen 905 percent since the '60s. With inflation, the increase is still a whopping 73 percent.
Home prices
Adjusted for inflation

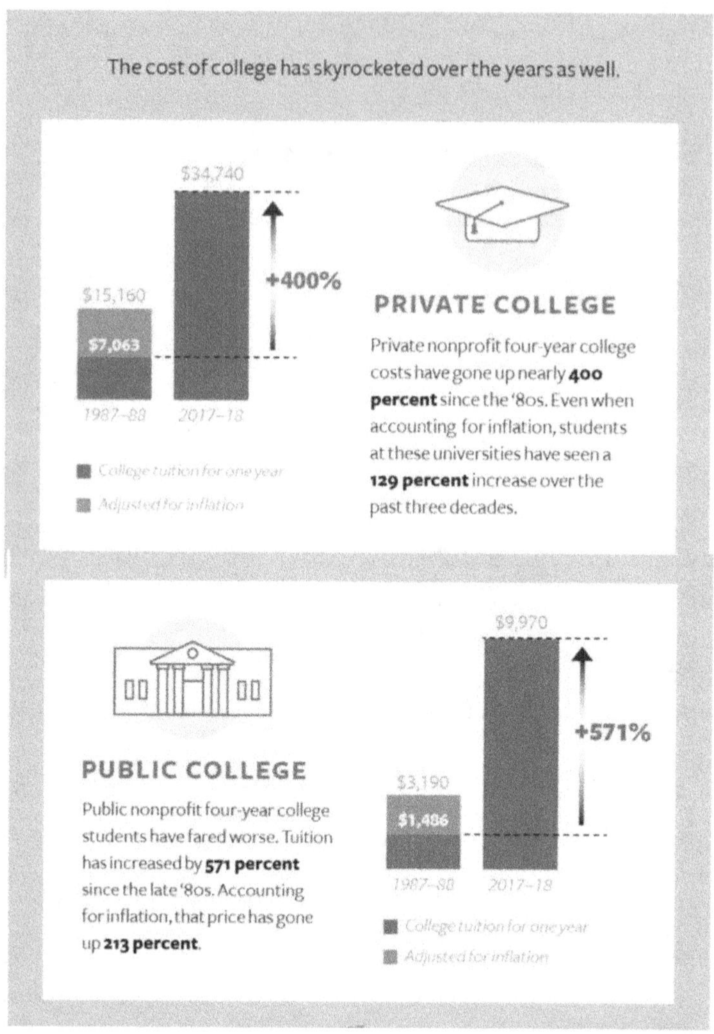


Because of so many common and often an excessive number of stressors nowadays, it is vital that those doing the Kelley program look very carefully at their lifestyles, minimize and delegate responsibilities to others that can assist, and prioritize what is most important in their lives so they can focus on their health and LET OTHER THINGS GO!

## Sleep Habits

This is an easier metric to quantify than "stress levels" as it is a more concrete "measurement" and less subjective. We can focus on a key measurement: 1) hours slept on average today versus forty-five years ago versus 1900. According to most sources, the trend is consistent—we are, on average, sleeping less than in the 1970s and considerably less than in 1900—by some estimates, two to three hours less, while other studies suggest it's a less severe decline but more geographically specific and circumstance specific, with those with higher incomes getting more rest and those more financially challenged often struggling more.[23, 24, 25] However, the research is getting clearer and clearer just on how detrimental sleep deprivation is to our health and how big of a degenerative stressor it is.

## Toxicant Exposure

On some levels, this is a more difficult metric than sleep, as most individuals have never been assessed for direct levels of heavy metal toxicants, pesticides, various chemical toxins, and so forth. So this, more realistically, is an inferred assessment based on some helpful inquiries into certain exposure

---

23   https://www.uchicgomedicine.org/forefront/news/2006/july/new-study-shows-people-sleep-even-less-than-they-think-whites-women-and-wealthy-sleep-longer-better

24   https://www.psychologytoday.com/us/blog/sleepless-in-america/201001/are-we-really-getting-less-sleep-we-did-in-1975

25   https://articles.mercola.com/sites/articles/archive/2015/07/16/average-american-sleep.aspx

trends, chemicals used and being added in the marketplace yearly, and incidence of drug use, alcohol use, and more. For instance, looking at the per capita rate of smoking, alcohol consumption, use of chemicals in the home, and pesticide use per capita can all be useful indices in getting a better sense of this issue at play for many.

As an overview of the subject, a couple of remarkable and shocking statistics stand out. There are over 84,000 chemicals currently in use in the US marketplace, and only 1% have been tested for long-term safety. Additionally, some 500–1,000 new chemicals are introduced yearly, meaning that children growing up in this era will be exposed to more chemicals in their lifetime than in any other previous era.[26] Furthermore, globally, the number of chemicals used is in the hundreds of thousands, with other countries, to varying degrees, struggling with how to regulate and control these.[27]

There are a few positive trends in looking at some of this data: Research looking at cigarette smoking and alcohol consumption since the mid-twentieth century shows positive trends in Americans' use of both; declines in almost all age cohorts have gradually been happening over the last six decades.[28] So the issue of where most peoples' chemical/toxicant exposure is coming from is not from some of the most

---

26  https://www.alternet.org/2015/07/84000-chemicals-use- humanity-only-1-percent-have-been-safely-tested/; https:// www.pbs.org/newshour/science/it-could-take-centuries- for-epa-to-test-all-the-unregulated-chemicals-under-a-new- landmark-bill

27  http://old.iss.it/binary/publ/cont/ANN_08_04%20 Binetti.1209032191.pdf

28  https://www.ncbi.nlm.nih.gov/pmc/articles/PMC2562028/; https://www.nbcnews.com/health/cancer/50-years-progress- halves-smoking-rate-can-we-reach-zero-n7621

traditional and obvious routes of exposure—such as cigarette smoke and alcoholic beverages—but rather more insidious sources such as additives and chemicals in food, cosmetics, cleaning products, and such that are harder to notice and be aware of. Yet, we must if we want to be well in an increasingly toxic and chemical-laden environment.

## What This All Means for Your Health and How Environmental Toxins Are Now One of The Biggest Threats to Our Health

In sum, this means we need to be much more careful about so many things in today's "convenience lifestyle." From portion sizes (much, much larger than in 1960)[29] to the quality (or lack thereof) of our food, the additives put into our food versus decades ago, to food growing and processing/refining, the lack of adequate rest, exercise, and more and more stress, and last but not least, the introduction of GMOs and the rampant use of pesticides and insecticides such as glyphosate (i.e., Roundup).[30] In my professional opinion, one of the scariest applications of these pesticides is actually as "desiccants" (i.e., drying agents) to bring grain-based products to market sooner. The shockingly high levels of pesticide residue in various breakfast cereals, many of which are marketed as "health foods" to children, are largely due to this

---

29  A very telling and illustrative comparison can be made by googling McDonald's meal/portion sizes from then to now. See the following link as a good example:

30  You may have noticed the recent omnipresent ads popping up everywhere in media about the use of Roundup and class action lawsuits against Monsanto for being linked to a variety of cancers.

process.[31] Thus many people are getting their first big doses of these noxious poisons as little children, which really is criminal, in my opinion. No longer do we have uncontaminated mineral-rich soil and largely pristine, untouched crops. Rather, things are being contaminated from start to finish…and they're ending up in us!

This is another reason why it's preferable to establish relationships with local growers when it comes to sourcing your foods, or at least make good connections with local health food stores with traceable products to know what is done with your food, to buy local and organic as much as possible, and to also, if and when feasible, even grow your own! You'll never have as much positive influence and ability to control your food supply as when it's coming from your own backyard.

While this is not meant to be an exhaustive critique of all possibly influential vectors on health, the above alone illustrates a considerable trend of a number of societal and historical trends that are largely stressing and depleting our health cumulatively over time. And thus, what may have worked in a time when we had fewer forces negatively influencing us in more recent years often hasn't been enough. Thus, the evolution of the Kelley protocol…

---

31　https://www.ewg.org/release/roundup-breakfast-part-2-new-tests-weed-killer-found-all-kids-cereals-sampled; https://www.ewg.org/release/massive-study-finds-eating-organic-slashes-cancer-risks

# CHAPTER FOUR

## Understanding Metabolic Typing and Its Changing Role and Relevance in This Work

In the original Kelley protocol, Dr. Kelley believed and iterated a central, important dietary theme to this approach: Different individuals (based on ethnic ancestry and where those peoples lived centuries ago, geographically in the world) had different nervous system "tendencies" when it came to metabolism. He categorized these into three main classes: 1), sympathetic dominants, 2) parasympathetic dominants, and 3) balanced metabolizers. And depending on these tendencies, individuals would need and thrive on different dietary approaches and compositions, and if you weren't following your appropriate, respective type, this would work against your health, eventually leading it to break down more readily and earlier on.

What these categories specifically referred to was basically the following:

1) **Sympathetic dominants** generally trended toward being more readily in sympathetic dominance (i.e., "fight or

flight"), and thus, if they didn't eat the right nutrients and foods, they could, over time, "burn out" this system through too much stress and overactivation, leading them into autonomic nervous system imbalance and disease.

2) **Parasympathetic dominants** were basically the opposite of the sympathetic dominants: they naturally trended in a more parasympathetic dominant state or "rest and digest" but needed the right nutrient and food blend to ensure they could keep in balance with their sympathetic system or this could also lead to chronic nervous system problems and imbalance resulting in disease if their stressors were considerable enough.

3) Lastly, the **balanced metabolizers** trended toward a more naturally balanced nervous system state with a more variable diet. That said, however, through too much stress and an overly extreme diet (such as going vegan for too long or a too heavily meat and starch diet), they could push their system out of balance and become stuck in sympathetic or parasympathetic overdrive.

You can see below in the following chart the respective nutrients and foods that corresponded to being high for each respective type. This chart separates the types into 12 respective groupings, and the closer they are to each other in the chart, the more similar the nutritional needs are. Conversely, opposite sides of the chart illustrate considerable dietary differences needed.

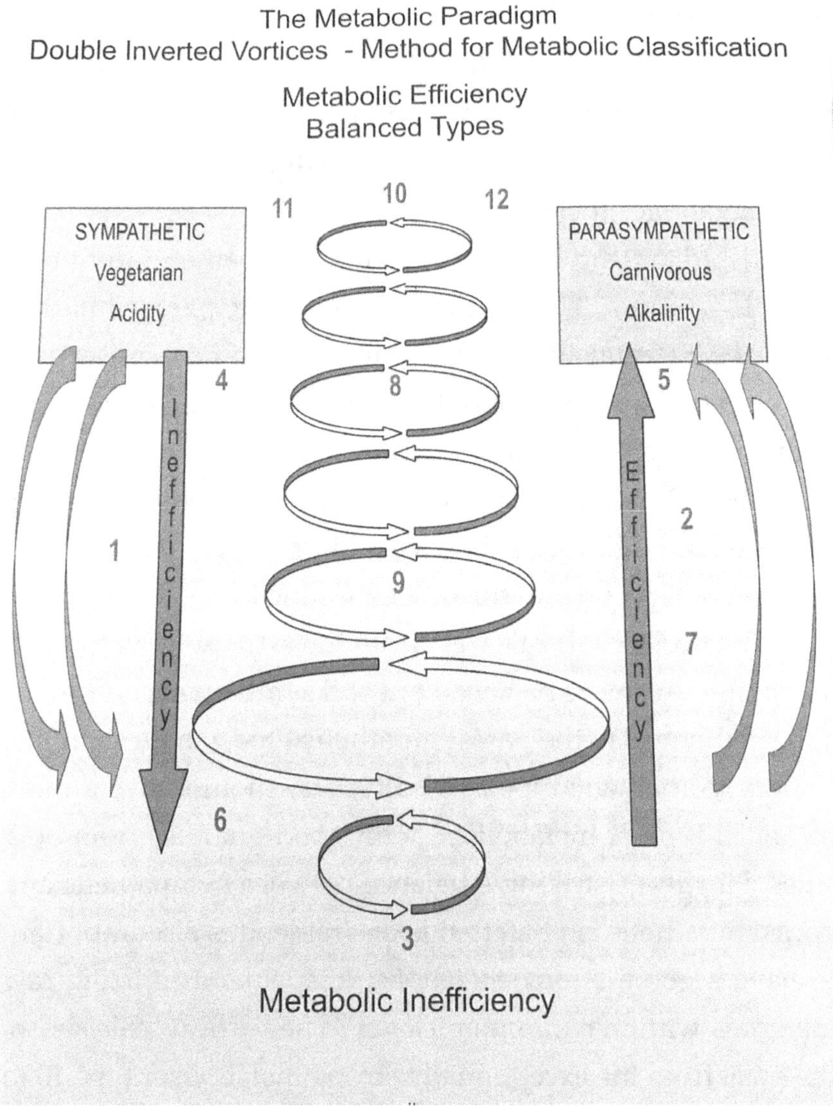


## Metabolic Type Spiral

Of all the forces of nature, the vortex is the most power-ful and expends the maximum energy. We perceive HEALTH and DEATH as two vortices. We cannot calculate the energy required to build health or the energy expended when one deteriorates to death.

This is what we call the Metabolic Type Spiral. It shows all 12 metabolic types and their relationship to each other, their sympathetic or their parasympathetic dominance and their metabolic efficiency.

Listed on the left side are the sympathetic dominant types 1, 4, 6, and 11. On the right side are the parasympathetic types 2, 5, 7 and 12. And listed in the center column are the balanced types 10, 8, 9, and 3; these have a little of both sympathetic and parasympathetic culminating.

These 12 types are arranged on the Metabolic Type Spiral on what might be called two sliding scales—one of them running horizontal and the other running vertical.

The horizontal scale runs from the extremely sympathetic type 1 to the more balanced but still sympathetic type 4, the balanced type 8 to the parasympathetic type 5 to the extremely parasympathetic type 2. Ideally, one should have a more balanced type of metabolism, with good qualities from both sides. However, striking a balance between sympathetic and parasympathetic isn't all that is desirable. It is also important to have a good, strong metabolism capable of utilizing raw materials with maximum efficiency. The vertical scale shows the scale from the exceptionally strong metabolizer type 10 to the good metabolizer type 8, to the poor sympathetic metabolizer type 6 to the poor parasympathetic metabolizer type 6, to the poor parasympathetic metabolizer type 7 to the poor balanced metabolizer type 9 to the poorest metabolizer of all, type 3. The type 3 metabolizer only assimilates about 10% of what he or she eats.

The objective of METABOLIC TYPING is to spiral from ill health (as in types 3, 6 and 7) up the spiral toward a state of optimum health (as in types 10, 11, and 12). This is accomplished by knowing that you are now eating the proper diet and taking the proper metabolic supplementation to achieve your optimum health.

Within these three larger rubrics (balanced, parasympathetic dominant, and sympathetic dominant) are smaller ones, as the above chart illustrates, totaling 12 metabolic types. As briefly noted before, these are all gradationally different from each other, lying from one end of the nervous system spectrum to the other. And thus, each diet for each respective type is gradationally different as well. Before beginning their work together, Dr. Kelley would have a patient complete a lengthy questionnaire (which is still available online for individuals to order and complete) to determine their type, and thus the diet that "fits" their type and should be what each respective person follows.

However, over the decades, Dr. Kelley discovered that this largely stable, reproducible typing he found in his patients in the first several decades was becoming increasingly less reliable and, in fact, upon repeat testing, was changing within weeks of retesting a given patient. Subsequently, over the course of many months of care, a patient could change many, many times, which made the test unreliable, as well as the diet very difficult for a sick patient to manage and keep up the varying alterations every few weeks.

Thus, as a result of seeing this more and more with an increasing number of patients, one of the most significant changes to the protocol was made, based on Dr. Kelley's observation of this increasingly frequent trend across many different cases: that the initial testing of metabolic typing was not done until the patient had actually undertaken the protocol for many months and had reached a relatively "healthy and stable" point of regression of disease and stabilization of many other health parameters.

In the meantime, the diet that was now followed approximated what was previously termed the "metabolic type four" diet, which was a fairly balanced metabolic diet—not too extreme in either direction of being overly sympathetic or parasympathetic and was found to work best for the greatest number of individuals, given this trending they were finding in case after case.

This metabolic type four diet will be noted in greater detail in the "nuts and bolts" chapter. In general, it consists of a very small amount of limited types of organic animal products such as free-range eggs, wild-caught and carefully sourced fish, and organic liver; lots and lots of cooked vegetables (almost no raw, which also surprises many people); lots of nuts and seeds and other high-quality fats; low-sugar fruits (i.e., berries); no grains; very little amounts of anything starchy such as legumes, potatoes, or beans; no refined sugars or processed foods; and limited sources of dairy (only raw butter [which I now caution to avoid due to generally elevated levels of polychlorinated biphenyls](PCBs) or ghee). It is generally "not fully" a ketogenic diet, although it can be easily made such by being more restrictive with the certain types of carbs allowed and rates low on the glycemic load and index matrixes overall. Overall, it is rich in fiber, low in net carbs, modest in protein, and heavy on vegetables and good quality fat.

This is obviously a considerable change from how the protocol was practiced in the first several decades, but as I mentioned earlier, science is not a static endeavor, and good practitioners and scientists evolve programs and plans when things are not working as they once did. *That said, the principle of understanding what helps to ensure good nervous system balance from a dietary standpoint and such testing for relatively healthier individuals is extremely important and can be done for individuals, of course, who don't have cancer as well.*

Two important concepts many individuals have not encountered but yet are really important to understanding the overall effect that food and nutrients have on us are as follows:

I.      The concept of dietary direction; and
II.     Sympathetic versus parasympathetic stimulating minerals.

## The Concept of Dietary Direction

This is the effect food tends to have on building, flushing/detoxing, and breaking down or generally maintaining equilibrium for the body.

**Dietary direction is divided into three directions:**

I)      Anabolic
II)     Catabolic
III)    Neutral

Anabolic foods are "building" in nature and specifically refer to foods high in fat and/or protein, both of which can build muscle and good fat tissue if eaten in sufficient quantity. Examples of foods that would be typed anabolic would include eggs, meats, fish, nuts and seeds, avocados, butter, tempeh, and tofu. These kinds of foods are necessary, to varying degrees, in everyone's diet to help with cellular repair and rebuilding, but when eaten in excess can encourage more sluggish digestion and slower bowel transit, as protein and fat generally take longer to break down versus carbohydrates in the digestive tract.

Catabolic foods are the opposite of anabolic foods in many ways. These are primarily fruits and vegetables that have an alkalizing effect on the body (there are a few exceptions that are not, such as avocados and coconuts due to their high fat content), as well as refined and processed foods (due to their sugar content, they also tend to "catabolize" or break down the body as well). Catabolic foods tend to have a flushing and breaking down effect on the body—often helping to rid the body of toxins, debris, metabolic waste products (such as acid residues—like lactic acid) and/or breaking down muscle (primarily refined/sugar-laden carbs). And these are absolutely needed in the diet (except for the refined/sugar-laden foods!) to accomplish these "flushing" tasks.

However, if eaten exclusively for too long, and not enough building foods are present, too much catabolism can occur, and the body can begin to use its own muscle and fat tissue to meet its omnipresent metabolic needs. If there is extra fat to burn up, this may not be a big problem for a while for some individuals, but in general, we do not want to lose muscle tissue for many reasons. Again—dietary extremes can get one into trouble!

Neutral foods, as the name might suggest, sit in between catabolic and anabolic foods in their effects on the body. They tend to have fairly neutral pH effects in the body and don't outright encourage catabolism or anabolism. Examples of these foods include whole grains and many root vegetables. If one is fairly balanced when it comes to their health (i.e., not needing to build more or flush more), then these foods may form a fairly substantial part of the diet for a given individual.

**Sympathetic versus Parasympathetic Minerals**

Many clients and students that I have taught are quite surprised to find out that different minerals have different effects on our nervous systems, generally speaking. Some minerals are more stimulatory, prompting more sympathetic nervous system activity, while others encourage more para-sympathetic activity. These generally can be divided into the two following groups:

I.     Sympathetic activating: sodium, chloride, and calcium

II.     Parasympathetic activating: potassium and magnesium

**An imbalance in mineral intake can further fuel nervous system imbalances between sympathetic versus para-sympathetic activity and is exceedingly common in the modern era of convenience and processed foods.** Much more common is excess consumption of refined salt (containing both chloride and sodium)[32] and, for some, excess calcium consumption by way of processed dairy or other foods.

---

32  Himalayan or sea salt, however, are much less processed and contain a considerably greater variety of other minerals, making them much less problematic and often nutritive for many individuals in many situations.

Much less common is adequate consumption of potassium and magnesium, which typically causes, in most individuals, an overactivation of sympathetic activity (fueling the stress response—fight or flight—which can be linked to why there is such an overprevalence of anxiety and insomnia problems, as well as adrenal and thyroid fatigue in Western culture).

It's so profound yet so simple that a significant part of this may come down to simply having a good mineral balance for many sick individuals!

## CHAPTER FIVE

# The Autonomic Nervous System: A Foundation Fixed via This Approach

    a. Mind Body Medicine—The Power of Energy
    b. It's Not a Laughing Matter: The Place of Laughter in Healing
    c. Positive Thinking, the Importance of Emotional Healing, and Optimism: Not to Be Neglected!

So, by now, you're quite clear that an important core underpinning of this work is to nourish and balance the nervous system by way of diet and mineralization and many of the other supportive therapies that are part of this protocol. However, by no means are the core elements of this protocol exhaustive in terms of what can be beneficially therapeutic for the nervous system. In this chapter, I will review several key, nondietary approaches that can be helpful in balancing the sympathetic versus parasympathetic arms of the autonomic nervous system. These include:

    I.    **The Wide Arena of Mind Body Medicine Interventions**—Some of these include meditation, yoga, deep breathing, Qi Gong, and Tai Chi

II.     **Laughter as Medicine, Nature as Medicine (e.g., "Forest Bathing")**
III.    **Positive Thinking and Keeping an Optimistic Perspective**
IV.     **The NuCalm Device**

I will also touch on the subject of emotional healing. While it is too profound and deep of a subject to thoroughly review and get into in this work, I will aim to outline just why it is so important and what some other groundbreaking doctors and researchers have found in this area that makes it so vital to address on your healing journey.

## Mind-Body Medicine

As mentioned, this is a very broad area with many sub-types of Mind Body Medicine, including meditation, yoga, Qi Gong, Tai Chi, and more. However different all of these practices are, they do share some unifying features, including focusing on the breath and calming and focusing the mind. They also share features of influence, meaning they can favorably impact the body in similar ways, including:

1.      Bringing the body out of sympathetic dominance (i.e., fight or flight) into more of a parasympathetic (i.e., rest and digest) mode. In general, this is advantageous for most people in Western societies, who so are often in a "go-go-go" lifestyle. A chronic state of imbalance between time spent between sympathetic versus parasympathetic state, over time, can deplete the adrenals and what we call the "HPA axis" (hypothalamic-pituitary-adrenal axis), which governs our ability to cope with and successfully handle our day-to-day stresses.

2. Slowing brain waves from a faster "alpha wave" predominate state to a slower "delta/theta wave" state. This allows the brain to also have greater clarity, focus, and less of an "alarm response" because it is not in a state of panic, which is too often the case in "fight or flight" mode. Interestingly, in a more relaxed state of mind, we also digest and heal better, and our immune response is improved.[33]

3. Improving circulation in moving pooled blood out of the abdomen into the extremities, facilitating better nutrient and oxygen deliverance to tissues.

All of these trends are highly beneficial for cancer patients in general, who, as we noted earlier, typically suffer marked imbalances in autonomic nervous system function. Moreover, they are all very inexpensive or free interventions that can be done, in some cases, anywhere at just about any time. This makes them indispensably useful, broadly-reaching interventions that many people can utilize right away.

For those unfamiliar, deep breathing exercises are often a simple and useful place to start. There are many different ways to do such exercises. One method I learned while in naturopathic medical school that has a long history in Ayurvedic medicine is something called "Nadi Shodhana," or "alternate nostril breathing." This is a technique that typically begins as follows:

## Alternate Nostril Breathing Technique

Choose a comfortable sitting position—either cross-legged on the floor (with a cushion or blanket to support the

---

33  https://www.ncbi.nlm.nih.gov/pubmed/25789375; https://www. ncbi. nlm.nih.gov/pubmed/15250815/; https://www.ncbi.nlm.nih.gov/ pubmed/27347892

spine) or in a chair with your feet flat on the floor. Allow the spine to lengthen so that the back, neck, and head are erect throughout the practice. Gently close the eyes.

1. Begin by taking a full, deep inhalation followed by a slow, gentle exhalation.

2. Fold the tips of the index and middle fingers inward until they touch the palm at the base of the right thumb. You will alternately use the right thumb to close the right nostril and the right ring and pinky fingers (together) to close the left nostril.

3. Use the right thumb to close the right nostril. Exhale gently but fully through the left nostril. Keeping the right nostril closed, inhale through the left nostril and deep into the belly. As you inhale, allow the breath to travel upward along the left side of the body. Pause briefly at the crown of the head.

4. Next, use the ring and pinky fingers of the right hand to gently close the left nostril and simultaneously release the right nostril. Exhale through the right nostril, surrendering the breath down the right side of the body. Pause gently at the bottom of the exhalation.

5. Keeping the left nostril closed, inhale once again through the right nostril, allowing the breath to travel up the right side of the body.

6. Then again, use the right thumb to close the right nostril as you release the left nostril. Exhale through the left nostril, surrendering the breath back down the left side of the body. Pause gently at the bottom of the exhalation.[34]

---

34  https://www.banyanbotanicals.com/info/ayurvedic-living/living-ayurveda/yoga/nadi-shodhana-pranayama/

Of course, there are many other ways to do deep breathing. A terrific resource on many mind body medicine interventions is *The Relaxation and Stress Reduction Workbook*. A perennially popular book in print since 1980 with many subsequent editions, this gives a beginner many options for deep breathing exercises, guided imagery, progressive muscle relaxation exercises, and more. Another great resource is the Benson Henry Institute of Mind Body Medicine, associated with Harvard University and Massachusetts General Hospital, where I was fortunate to get some additional training when I was in medical school. They have a repository of studies on the subject, as well as meditation and relaxation exercises, DVDs, and more for free or purchase. Herbert Benson, the founder of the institute, was one of the preeminent pioneers of the field in the 1970s, validating the power of mind body medicine through groundbreaking studies with Buddhist monks and observing the dramatic changes in their heart rate, brain waves, the ability to influence their body temperature, and more through deep meditative practices.[35] Candace Pert, PhD, also has written on and done extensive research in this area, being a forerunner in the field of psychoneuroimmunology. She helped to elucidate more of the scientific understanding of just how much of these kinds of interventions, including music therapy, can benefit the nervous and, subsequently, the immune system.

Specifically, the practices of Qi Gong and Tai Chi were

---

35  https://www.ncbi.nlm.nih.gov/pmc/articles/PMC2724877/; https://www.ncbi.nlm.nih.gov/pubmed/1801007/; https://news.harvard.edu/gazette/story/2002/04/meditation-dramatically-changes-body-temperatures/

crafted to "cultivate" and "move the Qi" of the body more effectively. For those of you unfamiliar, "Qi" (pronounced "chee"), is also known as "life force," the vital force that animates us and is present in all living beings. The practices of Tai Chi and Qi Gong have long posited that through specific breathwork, movements, and focus, we can center and strengthen this energy for health benefits. Anecdotally, many traditional Qi Gong and Tai Chi masters and avid practitioners have been noted for some of their robust health and longevity over the centuries, and personally, I have found these practices to be VERY helpful for improved well-being, energy, stamina, and recovery from adrenal fatigue.

Yoga is probably the best-known and most widely practiced out of all these mind body modalities. However, that hasn't always been the case. Before the last twenty-five years, yoga was practiced by a fairly limited number of individuals, and over the years, many forms and traditions have arisen, each with slightly different focuses and objectives. That said, they do all share commonalities, which again include focusing on the control of and mastery of the breath, steady rhythmic movements to encourage better balance, circulation, flexibility, endurance, and, at times, strength and a quiet, calm mind. There has been a growing body of research documenting yoga's multitude of health benefits for individuals with cancer as well as a variety of other conditions, including anxiety, insomnia, high blood pressure, and more. If you've never investigated or considered it, along with many of these other noted interventions, it is certainly worth checking out more seriously.

## Laughter as Medicine

We've all heard the saying, "Laughter is the best medicine." Well, modern science actually has helped uncover why there really is some truth to this. Laughter has profound, beneficial effects on the immune, endocrine, and nervous systems. Laughter helps to lower cortisol levels (the fight or flight stress hormones), which also, in turn, helps to lower insulin levels, which greatly influences sugar levels in the blood and can drive insulin growth factor levels, which, in clinical research, has been shown to further drive cancer growth.

Laughter, by way of lowering insulin and cortisol levels, in turn, helps to boost immune function, which is generally more suppressed when in a chronic fight or flight stress state. Natural killer cell and lymphocyte activity, notable cancer-fighting immune cells mentioned earlier, become more dysfunctional and depressed in a chronic stress state.[36]

Laughter also beneficially helps the body and nervous system by bringing the body out of sympathetic overactivation and into a parasympathetic state instead. Remember that healing and regeneration happen much more readily than in a sympathetic state and that nowadays, most people spend way too much time in a sympathetic state due to chronic, unmanaged stress.

## Forest Bathing or "Shinrin-Yoku"

---

36  https://health.clevelandclinic.org/what-happens-when-your-immune-system-gets-stressed-out/; https://www.sciencedirect.com/science/article/abs/pii/S0165178199001310; https://www.ncbi.nlm.nih.gov/pubmed/9251165?dopt=AbstractPlus

In the last several years, this traditional Japanese practice has been getting more and more attention by even mainstream publications such as Time magazine, as the importance of nature is being lost to many in our overly busy and "modern" lifestyles, and so are its many benefits. "Forest bathing" is not complicated; it is simply being in nature, connecting with it via all of our senses: hearing, sight, taste, smell, and touch. Yet its cumulative, regularly practiced benefits can be considerable, improving various health parameters such as lowering cortisol levels, improving immune function and circulation, improving blood pressure, balancing brain wave patterns, and more.[37] Furthermore, it's simple enough for anyone to do, very pleasant, often uplifting to the mood, and another zero-cost intervention!

## A Positive Outlook

We've all heard how important attitude can be when it comes to so many things in life. Well, it also turns out that it makes a considerable difference in longevity and disease outcomes. Clinical studies illustrate that those who report regularly looking at things optimistically, finding silver linings, and so forth, even in difficult situations, are more likely to live to 85 or longer and less likely to suffer from cardiovascular disease and other diseases or conditions "of despair" such as alcoholism, opioid addiction, and suicide.[38]

---

37   https://time.com/5259602/japanese-forest-bathing/

38   https://www.psychologytoday.com/us/blog/the-athletes-way/201612/is-shrinking-optimism-tied-drop-in-us-life-expectancy; https://www.independent.co.uk/life-style/health-and-families/

Maintaining a positive outlook can definitely be difficult when dealing with a serious situation like cancer, and many people need counseling and various emotional supports to help them get through this time. However, "reframing" situations and finding positives in what may feel or seem like a largely "negative" situation is SO important AND so helpful for improving one's odds of better outcomes.

This is something that can be practiced, and progress can be made for those who find this difficult or for whom it does not come naturally. And like many things, the more you practice, the better you get! For those looking for resources on reframing and changing one's outlook, please see Chapter 11 for additional references.

## Emotional Healing

Before moving into the core of this book, the nitty-gritty details of the protocol, I want to briefly touch on the very important and often underrecognized subject of emotional healing as it relates to cancer and health in general.

In working with more than several thousand cancer cases over fifteen-plus years, anecdotally, I can report I have seen a significant trend of emotional trauma and unresolved emotional issues in a significant number of cases. Certain pioneering researchers and scientists have gone so far as to suggest that for many cases, this may be the true key to unlocking healing in many cancer cases. Thus, I highly encourage peo-

optimist-life-span-expectancy-health-benefits-age-study-a9079206.
html

ple, at minimum, to seek out counseling support and potentially more, such as eye movement desensitization and reprocessing, emotional repatterning, recall healing, or a number of other related therapies.[39]

Given the surprise, devastation, confusion, sadness, anger, fear, anxiety, and other emotions that can come up with such a diagnosis, and then contemplation of what to do next, it is IMPERATIVE that anyone going through cancer care have a team of providers around them and certainly one, if not several, that can help to work on emotional trauma that may be playing a vital role in holding back their healing, blocking the nervous system from truly coming out of sympathetic overactivation, etc. Bessel van der Kolk's work on trauma and post-traumatic stress disorder (PTSD) has illustrated this tremendously well over the years. PTSD is more common than often recognized, and I've seen a multitude of cancer cases, more than would seem simply coincidental, where there seems to be a true link between where one's emotional state is at and its subsequent effect on the body's ability to maintain homeostasis and good health.

And lastly, one more tool to consider: NuCalm.

## The NuCalm Device[40]

---

39   There are so many possible individuals to mention here, but a
     notable few include Ryke Hamer, Candace Pert, and Deepak Chopra.

40   Disclaimer Note: Neither Pamela McDougle nor Eric Wood, ND,
     MA, have any financial or other affiliations with Nucalm. Our
     decision to include mentioning it is entirely based on positive clinical
     outcomes we have observed with its introduction into our respective
     client bases in the last several years. For more information on the

Medical technology is offering us new tools and ways to disseminate information and help to individuals increasingly every year.[41] One of the most recent additions to the core recommendations of this protocol has been to include regular, committed use of the NuCalm Device to help balance the autonomic nervous system.[42] We have seen profound shifts in a significant tally of clients in the last two years in regard to dramatically increased detoxification capacity, better digestion, better nervous system balance, and beneficial shifts in immune activity, which all add up to very significant positive impacts on prognosis for cancer clients! This has happened so significantly that after comparing results with our own individual practice clients over months, we felt strongly enough it should become an essential practice as part of the protocol.

Given the pace of life and how so many people are chronically stressed physiologically, it has made tremendous sense as to why this device seems to be making such a difference. Now this recommendation is not based on anything other than our own clinical anecdotal experience, but that said, what we have observed to generally work the best is to use the device for approximately fifty minutes in the morning before lunch. And for those individuals who have chronic digestive issues, we've found an additional fifty minutes after lunch to be very

---

clinical research, mechanism of action, and more, please see: www.nucalm.com.

41  See: www.healthible.co as a platform for helping to distribute and collate much of the burgeoning medical technology, apps, programs, courses, and more

42  To clarify, Nucalm is an downloadable app now that you can use with particular biosignalling patches on the wrist for greatest clinical efficacy. Again, see their site for more information.

helpful also. Perhaps someday, we will have clinical trial data to further elucidate how perhaps this remarkable technology can be best utilized.

# CHAPTER SIX

## Testing and Functional Medicine Testing: What to Do and What's Essential

As this program evolved in the 1990s and went through some adaptations, one of the key aspects that was incorporated into the protocol was the addition of key tests to: 1) better assess a patient's status before beginning all the nutritional supplementation and enzymes, 2) to periodically monitor their disease status/progress, and 3) to be better able to adjust their supplementation as certain nutrient deficits shifted.

The first test incorporated was one to assess the levels of **amino acids** in a person's plasma/red blood cells. Amino acids, the building blocks of protein, are key to healing damaged and dysfunctional tissue, and if a given individual is deficient in just one of the "essential amino acids" (i.e., one of the nine that adults cannot manufacture themselves), that will shut down the healing and repair process. Because so much is dependent on these amino acids, they have often been termed "rate-limiting amino acids," meaning if they're in short supply, they will limit the repair and production process.

I like to use the analogy of building a car. What happens if the assembly line runs out of steering wheels or tires for that respective car? It's certainly not going to be functional and work properly. Given that proteins are four-dimensional, if we can't properly "construct" them due to deficiencies of amino acids, that will truly be a big problem for their proper functioning in the body. And remember, proteins build muscles, organs, key immune cells and components such as antibodies, neurotransmitters, and much, much more—not something to be lacking in such a time, to say the least. Thus, this became an essential, early-on assessment.

We have found the best results of increases in essential amino acid levels into the fourth or fifth quintile on this respective test, ensuring that no "rate-limiting" essential amino acids are stopping the repair process from happening in clients. Oftentimes, MANY things are in need of repair and regeneration; thus, this is VERY important to ensure.

Secondly, as you know the importance of minerals to this protocol on multiple levels now, mineral testing has also become an essential cornerstone of early-on testing in this protocol. Getting levels of important macro- and microminerals in the body is key to helping to individualize the supplement regimen for patients and even helpful in directing them to focus on certain foods that may be richer in the respective minerals that they need and to minimize consumption of others that they are high in or are not in as great of need in. Incidentally, some of the most common mineral deficits we see today are many that relate to blood sugar control, such as chromium, vanadium, and zinc (is that really surprising given the current diabetes epidemic?), as well as magnesium, as mentioned before. Both of these tests can be ordered by clients directly via direct labs, or a provider may also order them, typically through Genova Diagnostics or Doctor's Data. See www.directlabs.com for more information. And while no test is "perfect" in truly assessing everything going on in the body and is always limited by the extant methodology possible in labs for such assessment, they are certainly beneficial and much better than having no data at all to go by.

For those unfamiliar, when ordering these kits yourself, you will need to get a draw done at a local lab center. Many hospitals, clinics, and lab providers, such as Labcorp or Quest, may be able to do this for you. Call your local centers first before going to one and see if they will do it for you. Some may; others may not. Those that do may charge a small nominal fee in the $10–$25 range typically.

Thirdly, an additional test set was added that looks at some key hormones, enzymes, and growth factors that may elevate or become out of homeostasis but are rarely assessed in typical cancer patient assessment. Research and anecdotal experience by Dr. Kelley, Ms. McDougle, and myself suggest these can be helpful to additionally check as monitoring tools in a given case.[43] This profile combining the consortium of tests is termed "the Cancer Profile" by American Metabolic Labs. As an additional "double check" to this test, in the past we have also cross-checked this test with the HCG test done

---

43  https://europepmc.org/article/med/91433; https://jcp.bmj.com/content/49/4/329.abstract; https://www.sciencedirect.com/science/article/pii/S0009912004001274; https://www.tandfonline.com/doi/abs/10.3109/07357909009012053; https://europepmc.org/article/med/8552208

by the Navarro Clinic in the Philippines, which for individuals on a tight budget, is a simpler and less expensive option alternative, although it has not been available now for more than one year.

## A Critical Note about Toxic Mold, Algae Exposure, and Biotoxin Illness

More recently, we have incorporated a crucial fourth functional medicine test to be done because of the sheer volume of clients we are encountering with this problem: **Mold toxicity!** There is a lot of confusion about mold and its effects. Sadly, I find very few physicians or laypersons as educated as they should be on the subject. Mold toxicity is NOT a strong allergy to mold; a person can have such an allergy from exposure or a predisposition to such, but mold toxicity is a very different situation. This is where someone has been exposed to a toxic mold bloom in an internal space that has "intoxicated" their environment and their body with various "mycotoxins" produced by the mold spores (these include gliotoxins, ochratoxins, trichothecenes, aflatoxins, and more subtypes). The most common contributing forces to causing a mold issue for buildings include: 1) a source of water saturating some organic material such as wood, drywall, etc.; 2) a closed space not allowing the material to dry rapidly; and 3) a faulty AC ventilation system, allowing water to pool on coils or other places, allowing spores to congregate and grow and "bloom." That said, there is a true multitude of ways mold can overgrow and become a problem in our experience.

Shockingly, nearly 40% of homeowners across the US are estimated to have had water damage at some point. Couple that with faulty AC ventilation systems, and many, many thousands and thousands of people are being poisoned by mold and don't even know it.[44] The chart below illustrates how big of a problem water-related damage is causing to homes, dwellings, and workplaces.

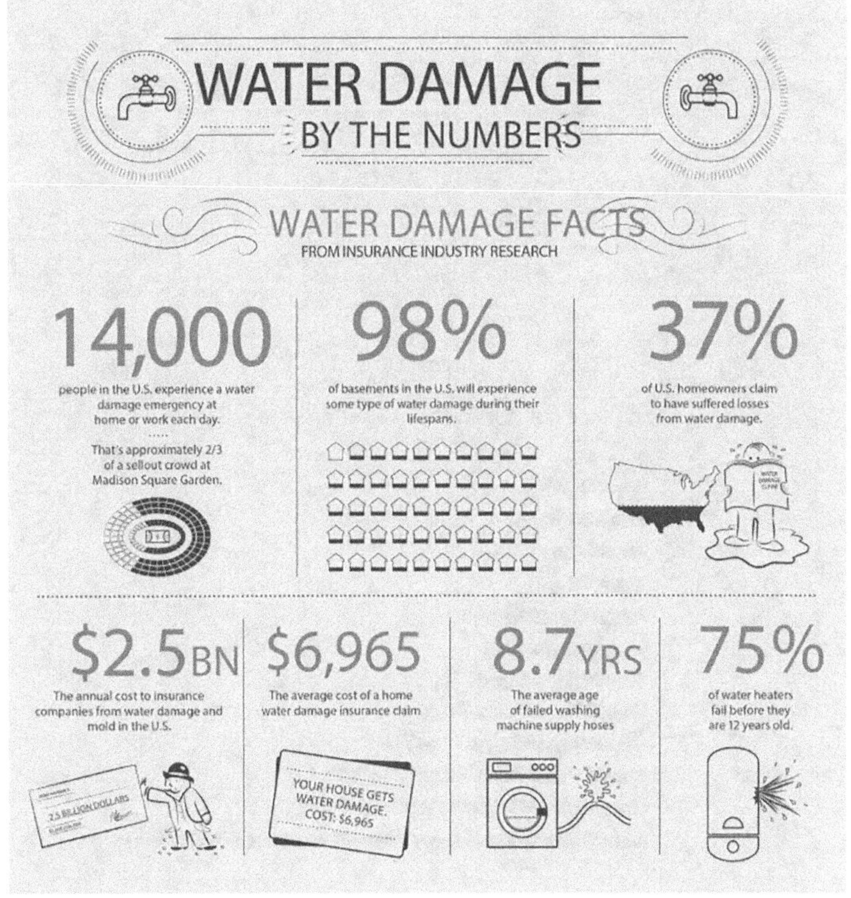


---

44  https://www.waterdamagedefense.com/pages/water-damage-by-the-numbers

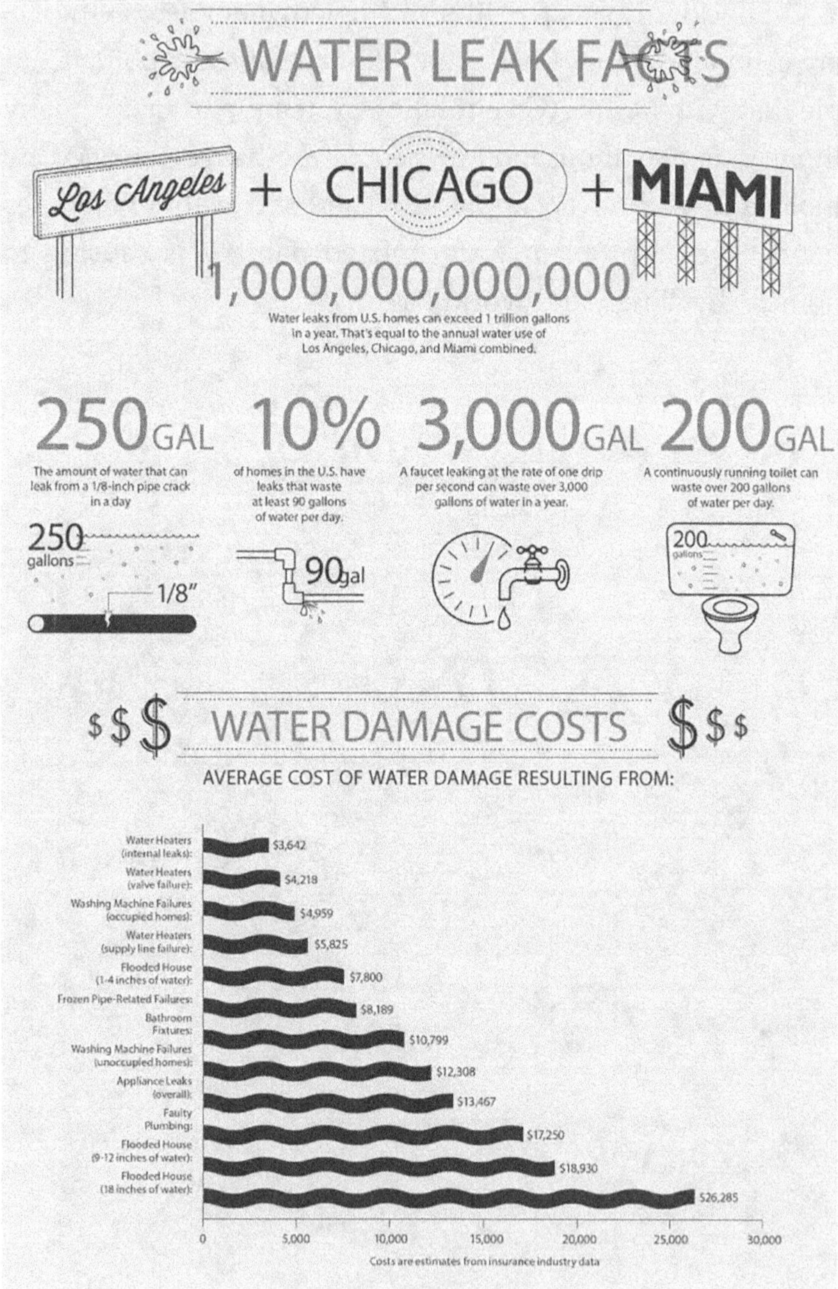
WATER LEAK FACTS
Los Angeles + CHICAGO + MIAMI
1,000,000,000,000
Water leaks from U.S. homes can exceed 1 trillion gallons
in a year. That's equal to the annual water use of
Los Angeles, Chicago, and Miami combined.
250 GAL
The amount of water that can
leak from a 1/8-inch pipe crack
in a day
250 gallons
1/8"
10%
of homes in the U.S. have
leaks that waste
at least 90 gallons
of water per day.
90 gal
3,000 GAL
A faucet leaking at the rate of one drip
per second can waste over 3,000
gallons of water in a year.
200 GAL
A continuously running toilet can
waste over 200 gallons
of water per day.
200 gallons
$ $ $ WATER DAMAGE COSTS $ $ $
AVERAGE COST OF WATER DAMAGE RESULTING FROM:
Water Heaters (internal leaks): $3,642
Water Heaters (valve failure): $4,218
Washing Machine Failures (occupied homes): $4,959
Water Heaters (supply line failure): $5,825
Flooded House (1-4 inches of water): $7,800
Frozen Pipe-Related Failures: $8,189
Bathroom Fixtures: $10,799
Washing Machine Failures (unoccupied homes): $12,308
Appliance Leaks (overall): $13,467
Faulty Plumbing: $17,250
Flooded House (9-12 inches of water): $18,930
Flooded House (18 inches of water): $26,285
0    5,000    10,000    15,000    20,000    25,000    30,000
Costs are estimates from insurance industry data

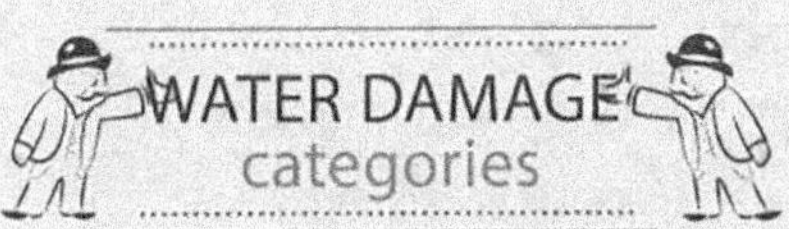


WATER DAMAGE IS CLASSIFIED INTO 3 CATEGORIES:

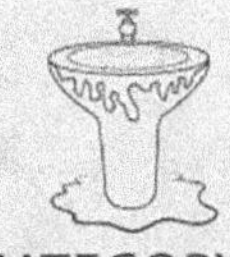 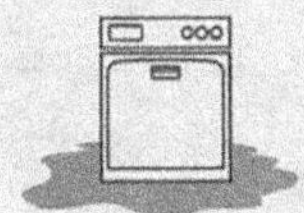 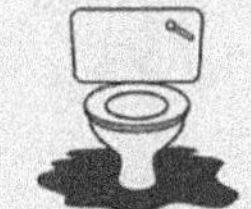

## CATEGORY 1 (CLEAN WATER)

Uncontaminated at its source and does not pose a threat if people are exposed to it. Example: Water from a sink overflow.

## CATEGORY 2 (GREY WATER)

Could contain some contaminants and might cause discomfort or illness to people exposed to it. Examples: Sump pit water, discharge from dishwashers.

## CATEGORY 3 (BLACK WATER)

Contaminated water, which could cause serious illness or even death to people exposed to it. Examples: Sewage spills, standing water, floodwater.

Note: These categories are not permanent – for example, clean water could spill out of a pipe and turn into "black" standing water.

# WATER DAMAGE PREVENTION TIPS

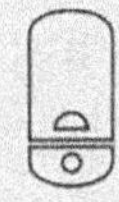 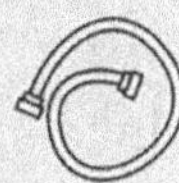 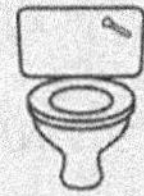 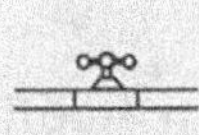 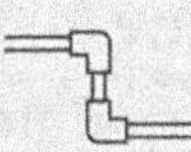 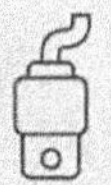

Have a plumber inspect and maintain your water heater on a regular basis.

Replace hoses on appliances like washing machines, dishwashers, and icemakers at any sign of wear. They're cheap, so replace them early, before the manufacturer's suggested timetable. Use the highest quality replacements.

Pay attention to your toilet - stay in the room until it finishes refilling. Get your toilets inspected regularly by a plumber.

When supply leaks occur, turn off the water - fast! Make sure your kids know how to do this too.

Pay attention to your plumbing system - look for signs of wear, including noisy pipes, signs of moisture on walls or floors, or rust-stained water.

Make sure you have a reliable sump pump and backup sump pump protecting your basement.

# WATER LEAK TIPS

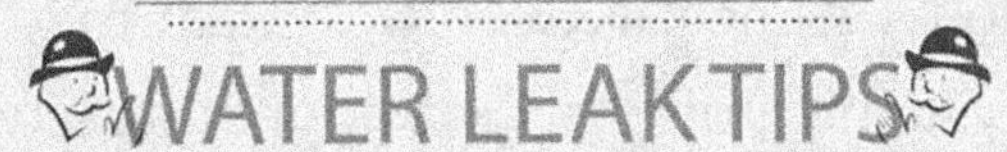

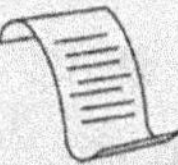 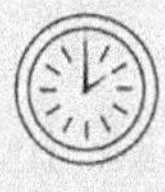 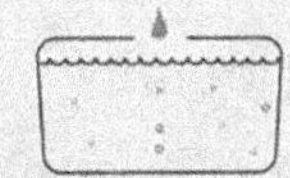 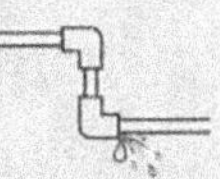 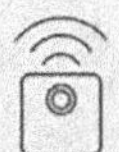

Watch your water bill for unexpectedly high usage. For example, during the winter a family of four probably uses 12,000 gallons of water or less per month. Higher usage could signal a problem.

Use no water for two hours. Read your water meter before and after this period. If the reading is not the same, you likely have a leak somewhere.

Check your toilet by placing a drop of food coloring in the tank. If colored water ends up in the toilet bowl in 15 minutes or less without flushing, there probably is a leak. Note: after you do this, flush the toilet a few times to keep from staining it.

Fix leaks and drips quickly, as soon as you see them. These are often quick, easy fixes that don't cost much.

Use water leak alarms and automatic water shutoff systems to catch leaks quickly.

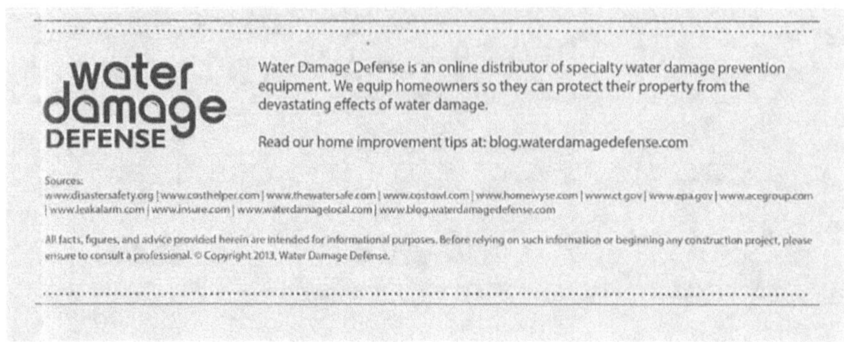


Source: Dr. Ritchie Shoemaker, Mold Warriors, 2011.

Incidentally, both Ms. McDougle and I have personally experienced mold issues in our homes over the years, and we know firsthand how troublesome, common, and dangerous this subterranean threat is!

Exposure to these mycotoxins can be extremely dangerous and harmful to our health on multiple levels. Dr. Ritchie Shoemaker was one of the first physicians in the US to start publishing and writing about the dangers of toxic mold (as well as algae) exposure in the late 1990s. This is due to the fact that such organisms produce something called "biotoxins," noxious chemicals that cause potentially massive dysregulation in the body. Almost NO body system may be immune from these systemic poisons, and approximately 25% of the general population is especially sensitive to these.

Below is a chart that details how many ways potential biotoxin exposure can cause health problems. Note that immunosuppression is one key side effect, potentially setting the stage for other increased immune-deficit conditions such as cancer.

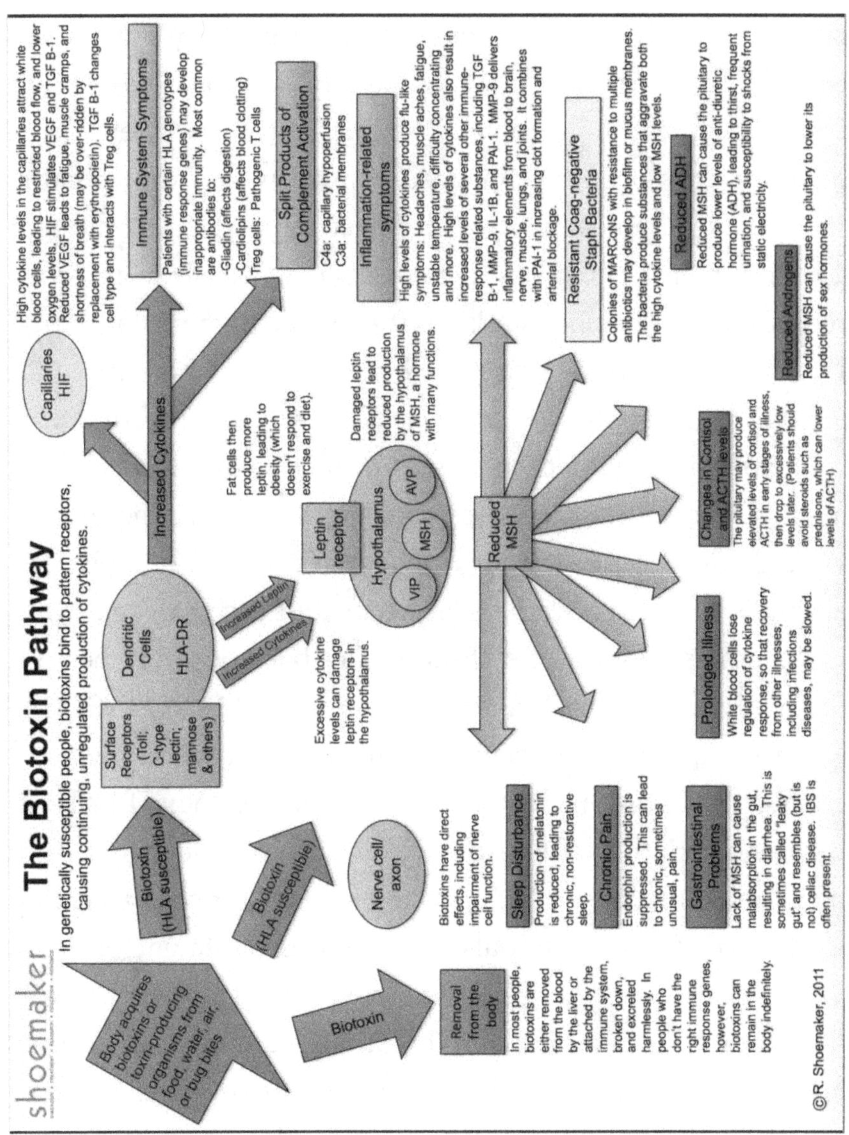


Source: Dr. Ritchie Shoemaker, *Mold Warriors*, 2011.

Given such stats, this is why this it an especially pertinent and worrisome issue for cancer patients. And a number of mold species produce toxins that can be mutagenic and carcinogenic. Thus, if we don't address this potential, often hidden cause and disease "vector," many people will not be able to truly get well; these toxins are VERY potent and nothing to be trifled with. Anecdotally, both McDougle and I have been finding more than HALF of our cancer clients have recently been testing positive for mycotoxin exposure. We believe it to be a true, underrecognized epidemic and paramount for clinicians to address if we wish to improve remission and healing statistics for cancer clients of all types. *We have yet to see a conventional cancer patient be screened for mycotoxin exposure in an allopathic setting, unfortunately.*

Specifically, for client assessment, I recommend looking at either the MycoTOX assessment by Mosaic DX, the Vibrant Wellness Mycotoxin test, or urinary mycotoxin testing by RealTime Labs.[45] All have pros and cons, but each can be helpful in the assessment process. If this comes back positive, then additionally, a nasal swab for what we term a "MARCONS" (i.e., Multiple Antibiotic Resistant Coagulase Negative Staphylococci) infection is also recommended via Microbiology DX labs. A high proportion of mold-exposed patients often develop a stubborn sinus infection, which this test screens for easily, helping to identify which individuals also will need treatment for this.

Additionally, a client will very likely need to screen their home as well as possibly their car, vacation home, and/or workplace for possible routes of exposure. Some of my preferred tests for these include either the EMMA test

---

45  Note: For very nutritionally depleted and/or stressed individuals (which will be the vast majority of individuals with cancer diagnoses in our experience), the best way to get an accurate result on such testing is by doing a large, provocative glutathione dosing (approximately 3.5 grams) before collecting a urine sample for the next six hours approximately, as the excretion of such toxins is highly dependent on glutathione and antioxidant stores to be able to process such through phase II liver detoxification pathways.

or ERMI/ HERTSMI-2 tests, available to clinicians for ordering. **In our experience, a client will NOT be able to recover from the effects of biotoxin exposure if they continue to be exposed** and are living, working, or commuting in a "sick" space. This is a VITAL point to understand if you yourself are trying to get well or you have the responsibility of caring for cancer clients that are "stuck" in their recovery process.

Please DO NOT underestimate how important it is to screen for and address this if positive results are obtained. We have seen unaddressed mold issues destroy health, careers, and family relationships, and that truly ranks as a tragedy in our book. This is a very specialized area of care that, unfortunately, very few clinicians have and one that both Dr. Wood and Ms. McDougle have additional training and experience in, largely due to necessity, both personally and professionally. Make sure you and/or your clinician have proper guidance in dealing with biotoxin illness should this turn out to be part of your case situation. We have both seen clients neglect this, and it ultimately was very detrimental to their progress and health outcomes.

## Testing Recap and Summary

**All of these tests should be run before a patient begins their pancreatic enzyme program.** Then, they should be done sometime later on, usually somewhere between four to six months after beginning the enzyme protocol for further reassessment, and every four to six months subsequently if they're continuing on with the program.

Lastly, after **every** full 30-day cycle, on the morning of day 31,[46] a routine metabolic panel is run called the "CMP-14," which examines some relatively basic blood chemistry, including liver enzymes and additional important markers like albumin, which can be important indices in gauging how one may likely fare moving ahead. Albumin levels below 4.0 may be more likely to suggest a poor outcome and may be related to one or multiple of the following, for example:

- Dehydration

- Hypothyroidism

- Chronic debilitating diseases (e.g., rheumatoid arthritis)

- Malnutrition (protein deficiency)

- Dilution by excess H2O (drinking too much water, which is termed "polydipsia," or excess administration of IV fluids)

- Kidney losses (nephrotic syndrome)

- Protein-losing enteropathy (protein is lost from the gastrointestinal tract during diarrhea)

- Skin losses (burns, exfoliative dermatitis)

- Liver dysfunction (the body is not synthesizing enough albumin and indicates very poor liver function)

- Insufficient anabolic hormones, such as growth hor-

---

46  In other words, Day 1 of the next on-cycle, but this lab is drawn before the enzymes pre-breakfast supplement routine is started up again. As soon as these labs are completed, the on-cycle is resumed that very morning

mone, DHEA, testosterone, etc.

Imbalances in lymphocyte to neutrophil ratio, ESR, LDH isoenzymes, and other lab indices found in such a simple test can help to further predict a person's stability or lack thereof with disease and enable a clinician to gain further insight into how best to help them in a given instance.[47]

## Further Testing and Considerations

These tests represent the core additions/inclusions of additional testing that Dr. Kelley and Ms. McDougle incorporated into the protocol in the 1990s, as well as the more recent mycotoxin inclusion. That said, for any given patient, there may often be a compelling need or desire for additional other tests that their particular case dictates. Some of the most common ones I have found a compelling need for, depending on the case, include:

- Circulating tumor cell counts

- Structural assessments by a chiropractor to assess impeded nerve conduction and other issues

- Comprehensive stool and parasite testing

- Nutrition genome testing

- Full hormone workup (e.g., testosterone, free testosterone, sex hormone-binding globulin, DHEA-S, estradiol, estrone, estriol, progesterone, TSH, free T4,

---

47  Johnson, Steven and Nasha Winters. *Mistletoe and the Emerging Future of Integrative Oncology*, 2021.

free T3, reverse T3, four- or five-point cortisol levels, as well as hormone metabolite ratios, including 2/4/8/16 OH estrogens and more)

- Heavy metal, pesticide, herbicide, and industrial pollutant and BPA/BPS toxin testing

- MRI imaging and PT/CT scans

- Allopathic tumor antigen tests, including CEA, CA 15-3, CA 27-29m, and a litany of others

- Genetic testing for cancer mutations (there is a long list here.)

- Liver enzymes and other metabolic metabolism markers, such as LDH isoenzymes and ESR, found in an expanded complete blood count or CMP-14 that have correlational relationships to health status

- Urinary hormone metabolism testing (especially important in those cancers potentially potentiated by hormones such as breast, prostate, uterine, etc.)

- Insulin and IGF-1 numbers, fasting glucose, fructosamine, HbA1C

- Vitamin D, B12, and folate

- MTHFR and many other genetic SNPs/mutations

- Screening for common latent, unaddressed infections, including mycoplasma, EBV, HHV-6, HPV (esp. subtypes 16 and 18), borrelia, and other tick-borne infections

This is not an exhaustive list but represents a number of the more helpful and often relevant additional labs that can be very advantageous to have in any given case. *Note, none of these are 'core program tests' and are not 'required' for doing the program.* However, many may have relevance and be advantageous in varying cases. So be aware and preferably have a team of practitioners to work with as appropriate to help facilitate ordering, review, and more. Of course, there may be others, especially given a particular case, that could also be helpful to assess. Remember, it's never just cancer that is going on in a cancer case! There are always other "clues" to dysfunction in other ways in the body if we look closely enough. Typically, many things have broken down and/or have gone out of balance in the years preceding the diagnosis that allowed the body to get to this point.

A good, thorough, experienced clinician will, upon doing a detailed intake assessment and conversing with the patient over time, get a better sense of what that given person may need additionally in terms of nutritional, digestive, detoxification, genetic, or other testing. **When in doubt, think like a good detective would and look for clues to help it make better sense!**

# CHAPTER SEVEN

## Breaking Down the Program: The Nuts and Bolts of Everything from Start to Finish—The Importance of Sequence

This chapter is truly the heart of this book. This is the chapter where I will detail the core of the protocol for you to follow, point by point, step by step, to truly do the updated Kelley protocol.

A couple of important tips: 1) In general, do NOT change up or substitute various products, other modalities, etc. for what is listed here. These points and suggestions are borne out of years of trial and observation, and have been found to be what has largely worked best for the largest number of individuals; and 2) When in doubt about something, refer to the troubleshooting section of this manual, or if needed, you can request a consult with one of our offices for further detailed suggestions and instructions.

Core components of the program to be completed include:

    I.      Cupboard clean out and stocking and household

product swapping

II.      HCl titration

III.     pH testing

IV.     Adoption of the Type IV Metabolic diet

V.      Liver and Gall Bladder Flush and Clean Sweep regimens

VI.     Twice daily coffee enemas and far infrared sauna sessions and other detoxification aides, as needed

VII.    Completing core functional/naturopathic medicine lab assessments (to be detailed in this chapter)

VIII.   Beginning incremental dosing of the immunometabolic pancreatic enzymes (upward to a maximum of 72 enzymes daily) along with other accompanying detailed supplements

In this section, I will lay out, step by step and systematically, how you will go about getting onto the full protocol and why it is important you follow the steps as listed, don't do shortcuts, etc.

## Step One: Getting Organized and Stocked

This step, for some, may feel fairly simple, but I must say, it is absolutely necessary and vital to do properly as it will save you a lot of time, effort, and stress, and will optimize the effectiveness of this program as a whole moving forward.

This step encompasses many little steps, which I will list and detail below, that will get you ready to move through the rest of the protocol much more efficiently and also make it so that you're not overwhelmed with shopping, preparing food, stocking and organizing supplements, not devoid of key things you will routinely need, etc.

What I always tell individuals is that the first several

weeks of beginning this protocol will be VERY busy, and you will likely feel overwhelmed. That is to be expected, as there are many things to be done and many changes you will be making. This takes time and energy, so be patient with yourself! You will get there. Taking it one day at a time, making lists, and checking items off one by one can be quite helpful so you feel like you're getting things done yet able to cope with how overwhelming all these tasks and changes can feel!

## Organizing Yourself and Your Kitchen Cupboard and "Detoxing" Your Home

To begin, *this protocol will require a LOT of organization.* There is no other way to say it. You need to be ready for that. That said, it is doable, and as the weeks go on, it will become more and more of a routine that you're used to. Keeping a journal or notebook for jotting down how you feel week to week is helpful as it will be very hard to recall everything that's happened or been changing as the weeks turn into months and beyond. Every year, more helpful smartphone apps continue to come out as well to assist with organization and planning, so it may be worth browsing these to see what could assist you!

In the beginning, organizing your supplements for the week or even a month ahead of time to ensure you know what you're doing beforehand is wise, especially for those of you who are working and do not have much assistance with undertaking this protocol. Consider getting little reusable nontoxic baggies, containers (preferably glass), or other ways to separate and organize your supplements for the seven times a day you will be dosing your enzymes and other nutraceuticals.

As part of the process, you're going to want and need to pay attention to everything you ingest, apply to your skin, immerse yourself in, and more, as nowadays, toxins are around us in more diverse forms and ways than perhaps ever before. Investing in a quality water filtration system, preferably six-stage reverse osmosis for BOTH your tap and showers, is really a must. The state of tap water in many municipalities is atrocious—laced with heavy metals, pesticide residues, prescription drugs, and more. See www.ewg.org/tapwater to search your own respective zip code for the toxicants in your municipal water supply. Inhaling aerosolized forms of such toxicants through steam in your shower or a steam sauna is yet another way you can errantly intoxicate yourself (for instance, the chlorine in municipal water supplies), hence the absolute need for shower filters. If you can afford it, invest in a whole home filtration system to simplify matters. It will be well worth the investment over time!

Ensuring you are staying well hydrated each day by taking your weight and dividing it by two, and using that as a basic minimum for ounces of hydrating fluids is key.[48] This figure is the approximate number of HYDRATING fluids you should be consuming daily. Most people are chronically dehydrated, to some degree, and this affects blood circulation and distribution of nutrients, lymphatic circulation, and

---

48   For example, 150 pounds/2 = 75 ounces of hydrating fluids needed
     daily for a given individual at this weight. Such fluids, on this
     protocol would be water, herbal teas, and green juices.

hence, immune function. Coffees and sodas, which you will be avoiding during this protocol, are dehydrating and must be subtracted, if consumed, from your daily total and compensated for with extra hydrating fluids.

**NOTE:** Fluids should be primarily consumed away from meals to avoid diluting important digestive secretions. Just have a few sips as needed to take supplements and lubricate food, and avoid major consumption of liquids at meals or chew food very thoroughly to make it very watery so you can take supplements with this and cut down on the fluid consumption needed.

**Do not use microwave ovens at ALL.** Instead, use a toaster oven or stovetop to reheat food. There is considerable research showing the damaging effects of microwaves on the integrity of food, potentially creating carcinogenic byproducts.[49]

**No deep-fried foods or GMOs**, and eat organic as much as possible. If you can consume all organic, still ensure you thoroughly wash produce with a fruit and vegetable wash, or make your own vinegar wash and become familiar with the dirty dozen and clean fifteen produce lists, which address the fruits and vegetables typically most and least contaminated by pesticides. See www.ewg.org/foodnews/clean-fifteen.php. I also am a fan of the site www.whatsonmyfood.org to screen for the most common residues on various foods to also illustrate which are most vital to purchase organically.

---

49  Stossel, Richard. "The Dangers of Microwave Radiation Cannot Be Ignored." Natural News and Global Research (Apr 2, 2011); Joshi, Amit D., et al. "Meat Intake, Cooking Methods, Dietary Carcinogens, and Colorectal Cancer Risk Findings from the Colorectal Cancer Family Registry." Cancer Medicine (2015)

**Avoid aluminum cookware and nonstick cookware,** and preferably use stainless steel or cast iron. Also, avoid aluminum-based deodorants and using glyphosate (i.e., Roundup) or preferably all pesticides in your yard and environments. Both of these are noxious, health-damaging substances linked to a multitude of negative health outcomes. Incidentally, be aware if you are in close proximity (a quarter mile or less) to a golf course, as they typically use copious amounts of herbicides and pesticides to keep their lawns looking so pristine. The air drifting and water runoff can readily contaminate nearby wells, yards, and gardens, so be aware.

**Turn off Wi-Fi whenever you're not using it, especially at night when sleeping.** Minimize electronic appliances in your bedroom and ensure the bedroom is as dark as possible. Purchase blackout shades and/or an eye pillow to minimize light intrusion.

**Purchase a cell phone cover or shield to reduce radiation exposure from your cell phone, and consider other newer technology to help protect your body from exposure too.** In recent years, a handful of companies have started to thankfully develop such products for personal and technology use, with independent clinical research studies showing benefits.

## Sequence of Tasks

It is important to note that many things must be completed before enzymes are taken for multiple reasons, most of all to ensure that sufficient detox and elimination have begun to prevent becoming ill from intake of the powerful pancreatic enzymes.

These tasks include:

1)   Completing the functional medicine testing AND the American Metabolic Lab testing

2)   Completing the Clean Sweep, starting the HCl titration, and checking pH to start correcting

3)   Beginning saunas and coffee enemas

4)   Beginning the diet

## Cyclical Cleanse Protocols—Summary of the Program

After your first cycle of supplements, on your off cycle, you should complete the "Liver/Gallbladder Flush." Once a month, on an off cycle, you will then rotate between the "Liver/Gallbladder Flush" and the "Clean Sweep." The details of both protocols are below.

NOTE: Before starting your supplement and enzyme protocol, you should complete the "Clean Sweep."

Sample Schedule to Keep:

Month 1: Clean Sweep Month (before starting ALL supplements, including high-potency immunometabolic enzymes)[50]

Month 2: Liver/Gallbladder Flush

---

50  At times, the Clean Sweep is done before the Liver/Gallbladder Flush and vice versa, depending on the overall state of the client's health and liver/gallbladder function. We have used clinical discretion in making this call with different clients

Month 3: The Clean Sweep
Month 4: Liver/Gallbladder Flush
Month 5: The Clean Sweep
Month 6: Liver/Gallbladder Flush

**IF a client continues the protocol longer than six months, this rotation continues in the same sequence. Some individuals with more advanced cancers, who are more depleted, etc., may need 12–24 months on the program for the best and greatest response.

## Liver and Gallbladder Cleanse

Preparation

For one week before the cleanse:

Mix ½–1 teaspoon of malic acid in 32 ounces of water or take one 600 mg capsule five times daily over the course of a day with ~6 ounces of water. Drink throughout the day on an empty stomach. Brush your teeth after drinking, especially if using powder. Do this for the entire week leading up to the day of the cleanse.

**Actual Cleanse—A Two-Day Event:**

1. Drink the juice of half an organic lemon in a tablespoon of apple cider vinegar three times before 2 p.m.

2. No dairy, oil, fat, or meat for breakfast or lunch. Eat food that's recommended only: quinoa and any steamed vegetables.

3. Have lunch by 2 p.m. and do not eat or drink anything

between 2 p.m. and 6 p.m. You will complete your food consumption for the day before 2 p.m., except for what is listed below for the flush.

4. At 6 p.m., mix four tablespoons of Epsom salts or for more sensitive individuals, approximately 1800 mgs of powdered magnesium glycinate in 24 oz. of filtered water. This will make four 6-ounce servings. Drink one six-ounce serving of the solution. Wait 30 minutes to drink water. Drink as much water as you like after 6:30 p.m.

5. At 8 p.m., drink another six-ounce serving of solution. Wait another 30 minutes to drink more water.

6. At 10 p.m., mix a half cup of organic cold pressed extra virgin olive oil with the juice of a fresh red or pink organic grapefruit. Stir and drink quickly.

7. Go to bed and lie down on your right side, and be very still.

## The Following Day:

1. At 8 a.m.—Coffee enema. Then, drink 6 ounces of mineral salt water solution.

2. At 4 p.m.—Coffee enema. Then, drink last 6 ounces of solution.

Note: If you do a colonic in the morning instead, you don't need to drink the salts solution this day.

Additionally for especially debilitated individuals: Some individuals may need to skip the liver gallbladder flush for several cycles if they're showing considerable signs of debilitation, difficult advanced illness, etc. This is best evaluated by an experienced clinician who can review labs, history, and make the best 'call' on the relative risk vs. safety of doing such. In such cases, the Clean Sweep is a safer and less complex intervention to do and begin with.

## Clean Sweep

**Materials Required:** Eliminator II (supplement available from Health Best Products); filtered water

**Instructions:**

1.  Add one level teaspoon of Eliminator II to eight ounces of organic green juice. Shake or stir to mix thoroughly in a jar or shaker, then drink immediately (the mixture will solidify if allowed to sit).

2.  Follow with an eight-ounce glass of water.

3.  Repeat this five times a day for five days: a) upon rising in the morning, b) before bed, and c) thirty minutes before each meal.

4.  During this procedure, follow your prescribed diet, but take the doses away from meals. Continue your coffee enemas daily.

When you have finished the Clean Sweep, resume ALL of your supplements and eat a high-quality, sugar-free coconut yogurt two times a day for the next five days to replenish your bacterial flora. We recommend only brands with *active cultures* and no added sugar. Additionally, double your probiotic intake for five days.

5.   The bulking agent can absorb many times its weight in water and enlarges much like a sponge does when exposed to water. The swollen mass gradually works its way through the small and large intestines, filling every nook and cranny. This helps to force out all the matter of stored waste materials that have gotten stuck in there that would otherwise not have been excreted.

6.   During the procedure, you may feel discomfort the first day or two due to the expansion of the bulking agent in the intestinal tract. This is a good sign and means the bulking agent is pushing out waste.

7.   Most clients on this protocol will pass many surprising things. Many describe passing long casings of sorts, like a snake or sausage casing that represents dried mucus, dead cells, and skin from the surface of the intestines. These wastes can accumulate over a period of many years and seriously interfere with the absorption of nutrients. Some clients with troublesome bowel motility may benefit by doing extra magnesium supplementation during their Clean Sweep and adding choline citrate, which improves magnesium absorption.

For those who have been struggling immensely with taking all supplements, we suggest continuing the following absolute minimum items during the off cycle:

1) Probiotics

2) Immune supports

3) Essential fatty acids

4) Liposomal DIM (if elevated/imbalanced estrogen values)

5) Liposomal glutathione (not reduced)

6) Continue enemas, saunas (with accompanying supplements), and pH testing and Pleo Alkala

7) Hydro-Zyme + enzymes with meals

## Mandatory Coffee Enemas and Saunas—Twice Daily

For more than a hundred years, coffee enemas were a recognized and important detoxification aid in traditional medicine until various forces contributed to their decline in use and popularity in the late twentieth century. In fact, they were referenced as a valid "treatment aid" for a wide variety of ailments in the Merck Manual of Diagnosis and Therapy until 1973.[51] Biochemically, they work to stimulate the liver and gallbladder to eject toxins and metabolic wastes into the bowel via vagal nerve stimulation by components of the coffee mixture itself, such as caffeic acid. This is why, versus just a water enema or colonic, they are much more powerful at helping "clean out" the body and why they have become a cornerstone component of not only this protocol but other -md "alternative" protocols for cleansing and cancer, such as the Gerson Therapy protocol.

Below are the tips we have found to be especially important and helpful to follow for clients undertaking enemas.

---

51  https://www.purelifeenema.com/the-history-of-coffee-enemas-by-dr-isaacs

These can be done at home quite easily and simply with the proper equipment and setup. In Chapter 11, resources for purchasing the preferred coffee, as well as equipment, are listed.

## Coffee Enema Directions

Typically, clients should prepare a quart of coffee using two tablespoons of organic green or very light golden roast coffee grounds per quart of water.[52] The water should be filtered.

Coffee enemas have been used for many generations as a generalized detox procedure. Despite rumors to the contrary, coffee enemas are **very safe** when performed as directed. Coffee enemas, much more so than just water-based ones, stimulate the liver and gallbladder to release stored toxins and waste, and this enhances liver function. Unless otherwise specified, we recommend each client take the enema each morning and afternoon, as noted in the daily protocol later in this chapter.

The coffee should be made in a stainless steel or glass coffee maker. Aluminum is not recommended since aluminum leaches out into hot fluids, and aluminum is a toxic metal. It is acceptable to make the coffee the night before to use for the full next day; this allows the coffee to cool and can be a time-saver for busy people. The coffee is best used at body temperature. If it cools too much overnight, reheat it slightly

---

52  We suggest Wilson's brand of organic green coffee. Green coffee has not been roasted and thus damaged due to the roasting process, preserving the highest degree of chlorogenic acid and antioxidants for the client's benefit.

on the stovetop before using, but only to WARM, not hot. When preparing to do the enema, lie on your left side, and lubricate the colon tube using "unpetroleum" jelly, olive oil, or coconut oil. [53]

Insert the enema tip (the smaller one of the two that comes with the kit) slowly into your anus and the rectum several inches in. Release the clamp on the silicone tubing and let about a quart of coffee slowly flow in, then reclamp. If the coffee won't flow, this usually means there is a kink in the tube, and you must withdraw the colon tube and reinsert it. At first, it may be difficult to retain the enema. Typically, you will hold the full quart (four cups) for 15 minutes. Do not hold longer than this—it is counterproductive. If you are unable to take the full amount of the solution, take half of it (two cups) and hold for ten minutes.[54] Then, release this amount and repeat with the other half of the solution. At first, you may feel slightly anxious or jittery, although most clients find the enemas relaxing. Usually, the jitteriness/anxiousness lessens after about the first third of the session. If you continue to feel more jittery, this means that you're making the coffee too strong.

After each use, remove all the tubing, enema tips, and connector. Rinse well with nontoxic soap and then add to boiling water for several minutes. Rinse again and dry thorough-

---

53  If there is a medical issue making lying on the left side difficult or impossible, lying on the right side or back can be viable alternatives that can still yield good clinical results for individuals.

54  Note: This may be a more common issue for people who have never done enemas before or who may have had bowel surgery. However, most individuals are able to gradually "train the bowel" to take more of the solution and hold it longer with practice.

ly. Let the silicone tubing hang to dry. **Do not store in plastic** as the evaporating water can foster mold/bacteria growth in enclosed plastic. Remember, you will be doing two of these daily during the entire duration of your protocol.

## Infrared Radiation (IR) Saunas

The other essential component of the daily detoxification process in the program is the infrared saunas. It's important to remember that sweating is one of the body's healthiest reactions. Specifically, infrared heat penetrates more deeply into the body versus conventional dry or steam saunas, thereby stimulating more profound sweating without the feelings of suffocation and the discomfort of more extreme temperature-induced sweating of typical, conventional dry and steam saunas. Research also suggests that far infrared saunas are much more effective at helping the body dislodge and excrete noxious toxins versus conventional saunas as well. In many countries, such as Germany, the medical application of inducing sweating via heat therapy (hyperthermia) is already widely incorporated into medical practices for a number of clinically validated reasons.[55] In the US, Duke University is one of the early adopters in this application for selected conditions and situations.[56]

Sweating from IR saunas produces these documented

---

55  https://health.clevelandclinic.org/hyperthermia-why-heat-can-make-cancer-treatments-more-potent/

56  https://corporate.dukehealth.org/news-listing/feature-duke-physicians-turn-heat-tumors-hasten-their-demise

clinical beneficial effects:[57]

a.  The sauna creates a "fever" reaction that helps to kill potentially dangerous viruses and bacteria and increases the number of leucocytes in the blood, thereby strengthening the immune system.

b.  It helps to excrete toxins from the body, including many heavy metals, pesticide toxins, hormonally disruptive plastic residues such as BPA, and more.

c.  It stimulates vasodilation of peripheral vessels, which helps relieve pain.

d.  It stimulates metabolism, often contributing to excess fat tissue loss and improved body composition (i.e., lean muscle to fat tissue ratio).

Remember, these saunas can be done in the comfort of your home in one of several ways. There are, of course, a multitude of saunas for purchase, but we would not recommend the vast majority of these. One must be VERY careful of EMF output as well as materials used in the construction of most saunas. Many conventional brands use toxic glues or other impure materials that can defeat the purpose of trying to detox in many cases! If possible, it may be best to build your own or have one built for you following instructions available in Dr. Larry Wilson's book Manual of Sauna Therapy. This can be obtained online via his website at http://drlwilson. com/BOOKS/saunabook.htm. When building your own, we specify a very particular type of bulb to use, specifically: Syl-

---

57  http://altmedrev.com/archive/publications/16/3/215.pdf

vania 250R40 Red Infrared Lamps. It's very important to use these in particular to get the most benefit with safety.

If it's not possible for you to build your own or have it built for you, there are a couple of commercial brands we can recommend of superior quality that you can purchase from by contacting our offices for further suggestions.

**NOTE:** *The light bulb sauna must be set up immediately at the beginning of the program before starting everything else!*

### Your Daily Sauna Protocol Instructions:

**In the morning:** Start with 20 minutes and work up to 30 minutes. You should work your way up to 40 minutes eventually over several weeks. For most individuals, the desired temperature range is 110–120 F. We recommend getting in when the sauna is heating up to get the effect of both the heat and IR rays, usually somewhere around 105–110 F if going to 120 F. Rinse in cool water in the shower afterward. Remember: this is all done before you have breakfast, as will be detailed later in this chapter in your daily protocol breakdown.

**In the evening:** This sauna is before bed and before your bedtime supplements. The same duration and principles apply to this sauna as the morning sauna. Rest 10–15 minutes after the sauna and rinse off in cool water in your shower.
**NOTE:** *For most individuals, the ideal bedtime is 9:30–10 p.m.; the ideal rise is 6:30–7 a.m.*

**Before you take each sauna:** Dose approximately one gram of high-quality, preferably organic and sustainably harvested chlorella. A product we like is the BioPure Chlorella

Pyrenoidosa, for example.

Also, with each sauna, you will be dosing 2–3 capfuls of electrolyte solution with filtered water to ensure you're not losing too many minerals as you sweat twice daily. We suggest using the product "Selectrolyte," available from Health Best Products. Remember to continue to drink your filtered water while in your sauna to stay hydrated!

**After sauna and during rinsing shower:**

- Skin brush.

- Use warm water rather than hot and consider doing a "contrast shower" (i.e., hot and cold) to heighten drainage and circulation.[58]

**If you are having an intense reaction or "healing crisis," you may shorten the sauna to 15 minutes four times daily.

## Foot Baths

It is also highly recommended to do daily foot baths, as noted below, to help with excretion. These are very simple to do.

**Items Needed:** Organic magnesium bath crystals (Epsom salts—available at Walgreens, CVS, online, etc.) and basin

Directions

- Put three big handfuls of the organic magnesium crystals in a stainless steel pan/basin with warm fil-

---

58  Generally it is suggested to do a 3:1 ratio of warm to cold water. The greater the temperature contrast the more considerable the impact, but ensure you're using temperatures that are not uncomfortable to your skin.

tered water.

- Soak feet for 30 minutes once a day, preferably before bedtime. If bedtime isn't feasible, then any other time during the day is OK.

## HCl Titration

1. If you have a history of active ulcers or gastritis, do not take the supplement Hydro-Zyme, which is the preferred product for doing the titration listed here.

2. After taking a few bites of food, when you begin your meals, take one Hydro-Zyme. After every three days, in- crease by one Hydro-Zyme. If you get up to six Hydro-Zyme without experiencing any discomfort, you should continue taking six with each meal.

NOTE: Five Hydro-Zymes equal approximately one Betaine Plus HP. You may substitute Betaine Plus HP for Hydro-Zyme if you are consistently taking five or more.

**IF** at any time you feel a warm feeling in your stomach or heartburn that you were not previously experiencing, stop increasing the Hydro-Zyme product. Decrease it to the num- ber of tablets previously taken when you didn't get this feel- ing and continue at that dosage with your meals.

3. Make sure to note your dosage in your notebook/journal and discuss this process with your doctor in your follow-up appointments.

*It is essential to correct low stomach acid production,* which we have found in the vast majority of individuals due to a weakening of the nervous system signaling, influencing the stomach's digestive output. Without good acid output, food is not sanitized properly from microbial contamination (increasing one's risk for food poisoning and/or intestinal infections), and protein is not cleaved into the right size for later absorption. Moreover, histamine complexes are also not broken down adequately, typically resulting in increased allergic and sensitivity reactions to a large variety of foods. **Remember, you are what you ABSORB, not what you eat!**

## The Importance of pH and pH Testing

Chronic diseases such as cancer flourish in low oxygen, acidic pH environments in the body, which are also, coincidentally, low oxygen environments. Hence, an important part of this program is testing and correcting pH imbalances in individuals typically driven by dietary and mineral intake deficits.

**Testing:**

- Every day, you will test your urinary pH shortly after rising. There are a number of companies that produce pH testing strips (and are available online).

- Take the pH test strip and hold it in the stream of urine until wet for several seconds.

- We desire a pH of 6.5–7.5 for the first-morning urine. For testing saliva, we have seen a narrower ideal range, in the 6.8–7.2 range, but we typically prefer urine.

- To correct a too-acidic pH, look at using a high-quality magnesium supplement or a mixed mineral powder such as Pleo Alkala "N," Basenpulver, or Tri-Salts. Depending on the level, the amount necessary to correct and bring the pH up will vary between individuals. Typically, this may be 1–1.5 scoops of the Pleo Alkala "N" powder in divided doses in a few ounces of room temperature water daily first thing in the morning and before bedtime, but this will vary between clients as well as over time in one's protocol, as mineral levels, oxygenation, circulation, and nutritional statuses improve in an individual. For a magnesium supplement, we have also seen good benefits from Perque's magnesium blend (aided by choline citrate), for example.

- As you move along in the program, you may not need to take this every day if your urine is consistently staying in the ideal range, which is typically helped by good amounts of greens and green juice.

- Consider taking your dose of magnesium or Pleo Alkala "N" before bed, preferably.[59]

### The Daily Protocol

This is the day-in, day-out protocol that individuals follow for 25 days, or each cycle. It is IMPERATIVE that this not

---

59  With clients who have sodium sensitivity that affects blood pressure or water retention/edema, we have substituted the two products Tri-Salts or Basenpulver N, with similarly positive results. On average, this tends to be about a quarter to a third of clients in our experience.

be lengthened, as individuals need the five-day break of the off cycle to ensure clearance of metabolic waste and debris. Without this break, it was often found individuals got quite sick as they were not able to keep up the breakdown ongoing in the standard 25-day on cycle. **This should be considered a MUST, and no exceptions are to be made in lengthening the on cycle.**

**Upon Rising:** (This is done once daily, approximately 1–1.5 hours before breakfast.)

- Prepare sauna.

- Take probiotics – It's best to determine how much is needed from stool/microbiome testing if possible; a minimum of 6–8 strains and 15 billion CFU count or more are some basic guidelines around choosing.

- Take high-potency immunometabolic enzymes (maximum of 10 enzyme capsules).

- Take immune support –There are many possibilities of various herbs and injectables based on the perspective/skill of your clinician. Do a full dose as listed on the bottle every time "immune support" is listed in this protocol.

- Take adrenal glandular (if the cancer is NOT estrogen-driven; otherwise, take an adrenal herb blend).

- Do sauna – A maximum of 40 minutes. Typically, start at 20–25 minutes and work up as tolerated within several weeks. This is dosed with Selectrolyte (three capfuls in eight ounces of filtered water) for replacing electrolytes and chlorella/cilantro for binding heavy metals (typically 1,000 mg).

- Do a coffee enema – As per the instructions earlier in this chapter.

- Amino acids – We have found the "Perfect Aminos" brand to test/work best. Dosing is determined based on the amino acid testing completed. Typically, dosing will run between 5–10 capsules three times daily in divided doses, as noted in this daily program schedule. *We have found this must be taken no later than 23 minutes before eating so the absorption is ideal/complete before eating food.*

**With Breakfast:** (Note: if not consuming liver as a food, two capsules of the supplement will need to be consumed as also noted in the dietary section.)

- EFAs – These are best determined by nutritional testing if possible.

- Vitamin and mineral support – This is best determined after amino acid and mineral testing.

- Hydro-Zyme – Take as dosed per HCl challenge for each individual.

- Plant-based digestive enzymes – May vary based on the composition of the meal and the individual but often 1–3 capsules.

- Vitamin D – Best dosed based on blood levels. D3 with K2 is considerably preferred over D2.

- Thymus Glandular – Take as directed on the bottle for

one serving.

- Calcium/Magnesium – Best dosed based on nutrient testing.

- ~1,000 mg of vitamin C (preferably liposomal)

- High-potency immunometabolic enzymes (maximum of 12)

- Breast Protect or preferably Liposomal DIM if estrogen (i.e., estradiol and/or estrone) is elevated on the hormone profile.

## One Hour Before Lunch:

- Immunometabolic enzymes (maximum of 10)

- Immune Support – A diverse number of choices are possible here, such as astragalus root, various medicinal mushrooms, etc.

- Adrenal Glandular (if the cancer is NOT estrogen-driven; if so, then an herbal blend)

- Amino Acids – Again, dosing based on amino acid test results. A maximum of 10. This must be taken no later than 23 minutes before eating so the absorption is ideal/complete before eating food.

## With Lunch:

- Vitamins – TBD based on nutrient testing.

- Plant-based digestive enzymes (1–3 capsules typically)

- Immunometabolic enzymes (maximum of 12)

- Hydro-Zyme

**Before 4 p.m.:**

- Coffee enema

**One Hour before Dinner**

- Immunometabolic enzymes (maximum of 10)

- Immune support

- Amino Acids – Third dose of the day, max 10

**With Dinner:**

**Note:** The dinner regimen is essentially the same as break- fast—an easy way for individuals to remember this. This also means liver capsules will be necessary again if liver has not been consumed as a dietary item. Again, see the dietary section later in this chapter for these details.

- EFAs

- Vitamin and Mineral Support – Dose this as dosed with breakfast.

- Plant-based digestive enzymes

- Vitamin D

- Thymus Glandular – One serving as directed on the bottle.

- Calcium/Magnesium – TBD based on the mineral test levels.

- 1,000 mg vitamin C (liposomal)

- Liposomal DIM or Indoplex (if elevated or disturbed estrogen metabolism)

- Immunometabolic enzymes (maximum of 12)

- Hydro-Zyme – As per HCl titration.

**Shortly After Dinner:**

- Sauna + 3 capfuls of Selectrolytes in eight ounces of filtered water + chlorella/cilantro[60]

**At Bedtime:**

- Immunometabolic enzymes (6 maximum)

- Spleen Glandular Support – One serving

## The Monthly Off Cycle

For the remaining five days of the monthly cycle, only some of the protocol will continue, with the primary exception being that **no pancreatic (immunometabolic) enzymes will be taken**. Continue with twice-daily saunas and enemas. To refresh the memory, remember the core off-cycle protocol is:

1. Probiotics
2. Immune supports
3. EFAs
4. Liposomal DIM (if elevated/imbalanced estrogen values)
5. Liposomal glutathione
6. Continue enemas, saunas (with accompanying supplements), and pH testing and mineral salt formula
7. Hydro-Zyme and enzymes with meals

*NOTE: The only additional supplement that is introduced during this time is liposomal glutathione,* which will typically be

---

60  In some cases where clients simply cannot fit in another sauna due to work demands or illness, this second sauna is less vital than the first morning sauna.

taken before bedtime and in the morning before breakfast. It is best to hold it in the mouth for 30–60 seconds before swallowing for ideal absorption (preferably liquid for optimal absorption). It can be taken with a very small amount of water to dilute the taste.

During this off cycle, the Clean Sweep or another Liver/Gallbladder Flush will also be done to augment the cleansing period of this time. The Liver/Gallbladder Flush and Clean Sweep instructions remain the same, as noted before.

## Maintenance Dosing

Once an individual has no active clinical disease, a client may look at transitioning to a maintenance program for dosing enzymes and other supplements. Initially, clients will reduce the enzymes by half once a clear remission state has been reached, and in an additional six months, they will reach maintenance dosing. Typically, this dosing of the immunometabolic enzymes is done one hour before each meal at four capsules, with an additional 4–5 capsules before bedtime. Some other supplements and detoxification processes may be continued, but this is highly dependent on the individual and what other health issues may or may not be going on, and is best individualized with the help of a qualified practitioner working with a respective client.

## The Kelley Protocol Diet

## Dietary Guidelines for the Kelley Program

### Important notes about organic, non-GMO, free-range foods and food quality

*As much as absolutely possible, ensure you do not consume any GMO foods and nonorganic foods. GMO foods have lower levels of nutrients and toxins that can damage your gut and impair your ability to absorb nutrients. Nonorganic foods (especially in North America versus most European countries) have higher levels of pesticides, many of which can contribute to cancer and other diseases, and lower levels of vitamins and minerals. Use the www. whatsonmyfood.org website to look at food residues to further elevate your awareness of this important issue.*

**VEGETABLES:** EAT AS MANY SERVINGS OF VEGETABLES AS YOU WOULD LIKE. THERE ARE NO LIMITS TO THIS. VEGETABLES CAN BE STEAMED, BAKED, PUREED, STEWED, OR COOKED IN SOUPS. DO NOT BOIL THEM OR CONSUME THEM RAW, HOWEVER.

VEGETABLES INCLUDE: Asparagus, artichoke, avocado, beets, broccoli, brussels sprouts, cabbage, carrots, cauliflower, celery, cucumbers, Daikon radish, eggplant, escarole, garlic, kale, green and red peppers, lettuces, leeks, onions, parsley, parsnips, radishes, rutabagas, spinach, sprouts (no alfalfa sprouts for those with estrogen-sensitive cancers), squash, turnips, tomatoes, yams (no sweet potatoes or red or white potatoes, however).

*–FERMENTED VEGETABLES:* These include raw, unpasteurized sauerkraut, kimchi, or other fermented veggies. Eat one tablespoon with each meal. These can be purchased at high-quality health food stores or grocery stores. **NOTE: It must be labeled as raw and unpasteurized.** Traditional store-bought sauerkraut is heated and doesn't have beneficial enzymes or lactic acid.

*– SPROUTS AND SPROUTING:* Besides alfalfa and clover sprouts in cases of estrogen-sensitive cancers, you may add any sprouts to your meals. You can also sprout the nuts or seeds you use, as sprouting increases the nutritional content and makes them more easily absorbed. If you are unfamiliar with doing this, there are many wonderful resources available online, as well as in book format for purchase, such as *Rodale's Basic Natural Foods Cookbook.*

**NUTS:** Almonds, Brazil nuts, filberts, macadamia, pecans, and walnuts. Seeds include pumpkin, sunflower, sesame, chia, ground flax. Eat nuts RAW, unroasted, without added sugar or salt, and ideally soaked or sprouted for seeds especially. NO PEANUTS! They typically have mycotoxin residues and are more inflammatory than the other nuts. Note: Raw nut butter may be substituted for raw nuts as long as there is no added sugar. Consider two to three tablespoons as one serving. This can be used with raw vegetables or in salad dressings. Peanut butter is not allowed.

*–Soaking Seeds/Nut Guidelines:* The soaking of nuts and seeds on the counter in a small pan for 4–12 hours in approximately a half inch of water will help to neutralize antinutri-

ents, such as enzyme inhibitors in the nuts, and make them more digestible. Smaller seeds take four hours, while larger nuts like almonds require twelve hours.

*Note:* During the soaking process, drain the water once and then reimmerse the seeds and nuts with clean water. Soak almonds for twelve hours and sunflower seeds for six hours.

**SEEDS:** If you like sesame, sunflower, or pumpkin seeds that are seasoned and crunchy, you can first soak them, season them, and dry them using a food dehydrator with a thermostat set no higher than 110 degrees.

**COCONUT MILK AND COCONUT YOGURT:** You may eat unlimited amounts of coconut milk and coconut yogurt. It may be sweetened with stevia. DO NOT purchase "low- fat" coconut milk.

**DAIRY PRODUCTS:** Organic, preferably raw butter or ghee is acceptable, although I'm suggesting to individuals now to minimize butter as it is typically the food most contaminated with polychlorinated biphenyls (PCBs) due to widespread, worldwide contamination of land and water where cows graze. Ghee may be a bit better, or stick with the other approved oils listed as a vegan butter alternative. Use in moderate amounts.

**EGGS:** You can enjoy 1–2 organic eggs daily. Eggs are to be poached or soft-boiled.

**FISH:** You can eat wild-caught salmon three times weekly or, alternatively, other small, wild-caught, sustainably raised fish like herring or sardines.

**LIVER:** Getting organic chicken or beef liver is a **KEY NUTRITIONAL COMPONENT OF THIS PROGRAM.** Each day, blend 3–6 tablespoons of raw liver with your glass of green juice or with freshly made tomato juice. You may cut up the liver into tablespoon-sized pieces and freeze. You can purchase frozen organic liver from your health food store. **If you cannot tolerate the raw liver, you may substitute it with the "Pure Liver Supplement" by Professional Formulas** as follows: two tablets with breakfast and two with dinner. **This is a key part of the program, so DO NOT skimp on this.**

**BEVERAGES:** All organic herbal teas are fine to include, and thankfully, more and more commercial products are coming out that "work" on this protocol that are sugar-free and artificial sweetener-free. Aim for half of your body weight in filtered, nonchlorinated/nonfluoridated water. Use this water for drinking, cooking, and enemas ALWAYS. Filtered water, especially spring water from a verified clean source or brand like Mountain Valley, is preferred.

**OILS:** Olive oil or flaxseed oil in small quantities (1–2 tablespoons daily). Perfect for use in salad dressings. You can use extra-virgin coconut oil as much as you like.

**SEASONINGS:** You may use a natural mineral or unrefined sea salt and nonirradiated herbs and spices. Choose organic seasonings when possible.

**POULTRY:** Poultry of any type is not allowed on this diet.

**RED MEAT:** Red meat, which includes beef, lamb, bison, and pork, is not allowed.

**SWEETENERS:** Organic stevia is fine to use. Flavored varieties of it are also OK. For those whose bowels are not overly sensitive, monk fruit and xylitol may also work well. Xylitol has the added benefit of anticavity properties!

**FRUITS:** All organic berries are fine, and frozen varieties are also fine to include. These can also be stewed to make a fruit compote/dessert.

**JUICES:** 2–4 glasses of fresh organic juice are allowed daily. *Juicing Guidelines and Tips:* Juices may include small amounts of wheatgrass, celery, all green leafy vegetables, beet tops, carrot tops, collards, kale, dark lettuce, parsley, spinach, Swiss chard, asparagus, bean sprouts, turnips, parsnips, and sunflower greens. This green drink may be sweetened with stevia. In general, avoid vegetables below ground and use those above ground due to their lower glycemic load/sugar content. There are many capable and quality juicers out there. Some individuals also may enjoy and find a food processor such as a Vitamix very helpful to make purees, soups, smoothies, and more on this program.

## Special Daily Whole Food 'Supplement': Frozen Cube Veggie Blend

This veggie blend helps to increase microbiome diversity. This was inspired by Dr. Datis Kharrazian. Consume at least twelve to fifteen different organic vegetables daily in the Veggie Blend, eating two ounces of the blend every day. Rotate the vegetables with each batch. Blend and freeze the washed veggies; we like to use the "Souper Cubes" freeze trays, which come in convenient one-ounce portions. Omit any vegetables you are sensitive to. You can consume these frozen cubes by adding them to your smoothie or add them to your daily meals.

| Combine small portions of each washed vegetable to your blend: | | | |
|---|---|---|---|
| Celery | Red Cabbage | Radishes | Yellow Beets |
| Brussels Sprouts | Asparagus Spears | Carrots | Broccoli |
| Kale | Spinach | Chard Leaves | Cauliflower |
| Basil | Ginger | Dandelion | Parsley |
| Cilantro | Mint | Green Onions | Zucchini |
| Red Beets (with greens) | Thyme | Rosemary | Snap Peas |

**CANNED/PROCESSED FOODS:** No canned or processed foods at this time.

**FLOUR:** While all grain-based flours are not allowed, those that are coconut or nut-based (such as almond) can be used to make a wide variety of baked goods that otherwise may be off limits, such as muffins, breads, pancakes, etc. You will still need to avoid adding sugars and other "off-limit ingre-dients," but with the plethora of "keto" and "paleo" recipes nowadays, many individuals can get quite creative and make a multitude of items using such flours as bases and then not feel as limited by the grain-free nature of the diet. More and more companies are offering premade foods made from such ingredients also. Look for organic, minimally processed ingredients.

**PERSONAL CARE PRODUCTS:** Many cleaning products and personal care products, such as lotion, makeup, deodorant, and more, are full of toxins. **WE HIGHLY ADVISE YOU CAREFULLY GO THROUGH ALL PRODUCTS AND ELIMINATE THOSE WITH HARSH AND POTENTIALLY TOXIC INGREDIENTS.** The Environmental Working Group is a wonderful resource that has a database that evaluates personal care products, cleaning products, and more that you can access and review for free by visiting their site (www. ewg. org/skindeep). Use this resource diligently as you organize yourself on this program.

Specifically avoid: fluoridated toothpaste, aluminum-containing deodorants, conventional hair dyes, especially dark colors (Naturtint or Naturcolor by Herbaceuticals are safer), and conventional makeup (Bare Minerals is OK. See the EWG site for other suggestions).

**This comprises the "core" of the protocol.** In the next chapter, we will move on to discussing the testing necessary during the protocol, when to do it, the rationale behind it, and more.

# CHAPTER EIGHT

## Troubleshooting: What to Do When You Inevitably Have Complications and Why Detoxification Is So Often the Answer

While this program CAN be done by individuals who don't have a practitioner or physician overseeing them, it is best to have a practitioner or doctor who is skilled in working with natural medicine and functional medicine to, at minimum, have as a resource if you run into complications from parts of the protocol while you conduct it at home.

Many times, when individuals begin to detox, they may not feel great early on because they are starting to unleash a lot of stored internal and absorbed toxins that have accumulated over many years. It is important to understand that this is a gradual process and to not go too fast. If you try and go too fast with detoxification, it can overwhelm the body's ability to process and excrete toxins effectively. Pushing through pain and other signs that the body is struggling is ill-advised, as the body is telling you via your symptoms that it is struggling.

Instead of pushing harder and further with detox, pull back and incorporate more detoxification supports until things calm down.

In our experience, some of the most common side effects, difficulties, and issues arise related to:

1.)     Stomach irritation from starting the enzymes or the Hydro-Zyme product. This is yet another reason why it is KEY to follow the dosing as noted and also screen for any ulcers or gastritis if there are ANY signs of this beforehand to avoid causing further irritation or a bleed.

2.)     Trouble getting comfortable doing coffee enemas. This can often be ameliorated by first having one or several done professionally in a reputable colonics center.

3.)     A detox reaction causing malaise, a headache, and/or fatigue from increasing the enzyme dosing. This may be termed a "Herxheimer reaction." Rarely do we know the full extent of the toxic burden, potential infection burden, and emotional/physical trauma burden of each person, so when you begin to work on this, **a lot can come out in a myriad of ways,** and it is essential to support detoxification to the utmost on all levels here. We have also had clients have a bunch of "emotional detoxification" happen where their moods are shifting all over the place. They may be extra sensitive, prone to crying, angry, etc., as emotions can become trapped in the physical body from a lack of processing, and thus, when we start to open up all these routes of detoxification, the backlog of all this may come "pouring out," in more ways than one. Remember the notable Dr. Candace Pert taught us all about the molecules of emotions and that thoughts can become matter!

4.)        Fear related to doing the liver flush. NOTE: We have often heard that some individuals may have done this before and think they can't handle/tolerate it. However, it has been our experience that **if the malic acid is done beforehand, as noted, complications are much less likely** as it helps to ameliorate clearance and breakdown of congested bile and toxins in the liver and gallbladder. We do not recommend doing the liver flush under any circumstances if the malic acid preparatory period has not been done. Bitter herbs and homeopathic drainage remedies (as noted later) in combination with this may also help too.

Some overall tips we can suggest for helping some of these most common reactions include:

1.        If you're feeling toxic/fatigued: First, try doing an extra coffee enema and sauna or two and take some extra CoQ10 and vitamin C (liposomal). The majority of the time, this will do the trick and help the situation dramatically. Also, do an alternating shower with skin brushing (as detailed later in the chapter).

**If you are having an intense reaction or "healing crisis," you may shorten the sauna to fifteen minutes, four times daily.

- Also, consider doing an extra Epsom salt or vinegar bath followed by a castor oil pack and a short nap if you are still not feeling well. Practice deep breathing exercises, use your NuCalm app, and consider getting The Relaxation and Stress Reduction Workbook, as mentioned before, to review many stress reduction techniques. Remember, we detox and heal best when the parasympathetic mode is active, not when we are overly stressed. Also, ensure that one is getting optimal amounts of sleep (8–9 or possibly more hours) during these times.

- Milk thistle, oral liposomal glutathione, glutathione suppositories, as well as homeopathic drainage complexes by companies such as Unda, Pekana, Byron White, or others, will additionally support detoxification and clearance. There are many reputable possibilities here for help.

- Bitter vegetables, dandelion, milk thistle, and a wide array of other herbal teas can also be very supportive for the liver detox process. Use these liberally. There are also some wonderful traditional Chinese medicine herbs that can be utilized with great success for this too.

- Boosting antioxidant consumption. Some of the detox reactions can be related to inflammation brought on by toxins being released and injuring bodily tissues (which is part of what happens in a Herxheimer reaction). Some of our favorites to counter this include astaxanthin, CoQ10, R-lipoic acid, glutathione, and vitamin C (preferably liposomal or a high-quality formula such as those made by Perque).

2.     If the problem relates to stomach irritation, consider:

Using demulcent herbs such as marshmallow, slippery

elm, deglycyrrhizinated licorice, and aloe, as well as gut-healing nutrients and foods such as vitamin A, bone broth, and cabbage juice, can be very helpful in most cases to get the stomach to calm down. Additionally, if needed, natural pain relievers such as white willow, ginger, full-spectrum CBD oil, and others can all help in different ways to assuage issues in this department.

If the pain/irritation continues or worsens, an individual may need to temporarily stop the Hydro-Zyme and immunometabolic enzymes until things improve and possibly get imaging done of the stomach to screen for more serious issues such as a hiatal hernia, ulcer, or gastritis. In the meantime, one tablespoon per meal of organic apple cider vinegar may work as a gentler alternative.

3.      If related to coffee enemas:

Very rarely is the problem actually related to the coffee enemas themselves causing problems (although this is possible if there is a fissure, recent bowel surgery, or overly active hemorrhoids. In such cases, addressing these are key to ensure enemas are done as directed and appropriate). Usually, it is related to anxiety about doing them due to unfamiliarity for individuals. This is typically easily addressed by reviewing instructions repeatedly, potentially having one or several done professionally to feel what it is like, and also having a partner, friend, or a close family member assist in helping to do the first several until you get the hang of it. If hemorrhoids are bothersome, there are a variety of supplements, over-the-counter creams, and other devices, such as the Anurex tube, that can be very helpful in calming them down.

When in doubt, always consult with your qualified healthcare provider or our offices for further assistance if you are "stuck." However, for the vast majority of problems, we've found these simple tips to improve and fix most issues.

## Additional Detoxification Methods

In our overly busy, modern, and distracted lifestyles, we have largely forgotten a lot of the wonderful detoxification and hydrotherapy practices that, for hundreds if not thousands of years, many cultures have practiced around the world. The tradition of using water as a "medicinal application" (hydrotherapy) still remains especially strong in parts of Central Europe and parts of Eastern Asia, such as Korea.

Below are various additional detoxification aids one can use if someone is experiencing signs of toxicity, a Herxheimer reaction, or overall malaise and low energy to help the body better clear out metabolic toxins and more that may be being released while doing this protocol.

1.   **Salt and Soda Baths:** During periods of intense toxicity, a warm bath with added baking soda and salt can greatly help mobilize toxins out of the body through the skin. In a fairly warm bath, add one

cup of baking soda (sodium bicarbonate) and one cup of regular table salt (or sea salt). Lie in the bath for 20–30 minutes. Rinse with plain water when finished soaking to prevent the salt from drying out the skin. The bath should be repeated daily until symptoms diminish.

2. **Vinegar Baths:** Take vinegar baths at least twice each week. In a warm bath, add one cup of organic apple cider vinegar. Lie in the bath for 20–30 minutes. The vinegar will help to pull toxins from the skin. During periods of intense toxicity, the vinegar bath can be done daily.

3. **Mustard Foot Soaks:** This particular remedy is very helpful for toxic headaches, generalized "goopy" toxic symptoms, muscle aches and pains, and water retention in the ankles or other parts of the body. In a basin of warm water, add one tablespoon of dry mustard and one teaspoon of cayenne pepper. Sit in a comfy chair and soak your feet in the basin for 20–30 minutes. The mustard soaks can be repeated 2–3 times each day and should be continued during periods of intense toxicity.

4. **Castor Oil Compresses:** This old folk remedy works remarkably well to draw out toxins from the body. The compresses are particularly useful when applied to areas of pain where tumors might be breaking down. Buy castor oil from your health food store, pharmacy, or online.

**Background:** The castor bean (Oleum ricini) is known principally as a cathartic (strong laxative). As a pack is placed over the abdomen, usually with heat applied, the oil is absorbed into the lymphatic circulation to provide a soothing, cleansing, and nutritive treatment.

**Use:** The castor oil "pack" is helpful for the following issues: uterine fibroids, ovarian cysts, headaches, liver disorders, constipation, intestinal disorders, gallbladder inflammation or stones, conditions with poor elimination, nighttime urinary frequency, and inflamed joints.

**Contraindications (avoid using in):** pregnancy, over the lower abdomen with concurrent heavy menstrual flow, or the presence of internal bleeding.

**Materials Needed:** organic castor oil, a sheet of plastic, such as a garbage bag, a piece of cotton flannel approximately 36″ x 18″, a hot water bottle or heating pad, pillows, and baking soda.

**Procedure:** 1. Fold flannel into three layers to fit over the entire abdomen. 2. Soak the flannel with castor oil. Fold the flannel in half and strip excess oil from the flannel 'pack'. Unfold. 3. Lie on your back with your feet elevated (use of a pillow under the knees and feet works well), placing the oil-soaked flannel over the abdomen or the liver area (under the right side of the ribs), cover with a small sheet of plastic and then an old towel. Place a hot water bottle or heating pad on top to deepen its beneficial effects. 4. Leave pack on for 45–60 minutes. Practice relaxation breathing by placing one hand on your diaphragm and the other hand on your lower abdomen. As you breathe in, force your lower abdomen to swell like a balloon. With each breath out, practice relaxing your jaw and shoulders. As your practice more, relax all the muscles in your body. 5. To remove the oil, wash with a solution of two tablespoons of baking soda to one quart of water or a natural soap (such as Castille, Biokleen citrus soap, or African black soap). 6. Store the castor pack in the fridge in a large Ziplock bag. Add more oil only as needed to keep the pack saturated.

Replace the pack after it begins to change color. 7. For maximum effectiveness, apply the pack as often as possible, at least four consecutive days per week for at least 4–6 weeks. Daily use provides the most beneficial effects.

**ALTERNATIVE METHOD:** Apply the castor oil directly to your abdomen without the flannel pack. A sheet of plastic covers the oil-soaked skin with a towel on top. A hot water bottle or heating pad is applied. This is often applied for the entire night, and in the morning, the castor oil will be totally absorbed through the skin. This is the best method for young children. Use old sheets as the castor oil permanently stains. Keep the compress in place for at least 20 minutes, up to 60–90 minutes.

**The castor oil packs can be applied AS OFTEN as you need, as they're not harmful. BE CAREFUL not to overheat the oil so you don't burn yourself when applying it to the skin.

5.        **Skin brushing and alternating showers:** Skin brushing is a method of stimulating and cleansing the lymphatic system and detoxifying the skin. However simple it may sound, it is a very powerfully effective technique, especially when combined with alternating showers. Use a long-handled, soft bristle brush (with natural vegetable bristles) or a loofah sponge; these are available online and in many health food stores. The brush/sponge should be kept dry. The body should be dry, and the brush should be passed over the skin in a clean, circular, sweeping motion, not back-and-forth or scrubbing motions. Light brushing is best, not heavy scrubbing.

The brushing should be done starting at the extremities and moving toward the central trunk near the heart/lungs. There is no need to brush the face. Do this before getting in the shower, where you will alternate between warm/hot and cool/cold in a 3:1 ratio several times before concluding your shower. For instance, 90 seconds warm/hot, 30 seconds cool/cold, and then repeat 3–5 times. Always finish with cool/ cold, and wrap in a warm, comfy towel. In times of intense toxicity, the brushing and showers can be increased to four times daily.

6.      **Bentonite enema:** During periods of intense toxicity, another valuable aid is the bentonite enema. A single one-quart bentonite enema should be done once a week instead of your usual coffee enemas. To do the enema, add four ounces (1/2 cup) of the liquid bentonite to 28 ounces of filtered warm water to produce a quart of liquid. Insert the entire quart as a single enema and hold for ten minutes, then expel. Again, this should be done only once a week. The bentonite very effectively draws out toxins from the intestinal tract. This can be done after a session of coffee enemas but not immediately before them, as the coffee will wash out the bentonite.

7.      **Oil Soaks:** The body uses four main systems to excrete waste materials: the liver and the intestines, the kidneys, the lungs, and the skin. Too often, we forget to use the skin to help detox the body and speed the removal of metabolic waste. On this program, cancer breakdown products and other metabolic debris tend to accumulate rapidly, and often, our patients develop all manner of skin eruptions and blemishes.

Such conditions may be worrisome but should be viewed as a good sign.[61]

Instructions: *Once weekly, rub skin from head to foot with a mixture of equal parts of olive and castor oils (castor oil is available at pharmacies like Walgreens, etc.). With the oil still intact on the skin, take a warm bath for fifteen minutes. The bath allows the oil to penetrate to the deepest level of the skin. After the bath, get into bed under heavy covers for one hour to sweat out the toxins. Be careful getting in and out of the tub, as the oil will make things slippery. Finally, take a hot shower to finish. The oil soaks should be done weekly for the first three months of the program. At that time, they can be discontinued.*

If someone is still really struggling after considering and implementing all of these points, they may require more intense support, such as IV glutathione and/or temporarily reducing or stopping their enzyme protocol. It's best to contact your qualified practitioner or one of our offices for additional tips and guidance as needed.

## A Note on Combining Other Nutritional or Treatment Therapies with Enzymes

In general, many other therapies can often be combined with pancreatic enzymes without any direct contraindications. These could include oxygenation therapies, mistletoe

---

61  If someone must travel on their protocol and they're not able to do their sauna, some of these other detox therapies can be done as a next best option during that time. We don't recommend any extended trips while doing the full protocol for obvious reasons, however

therapy, Poly-MVA, hyperthermia, a myriad of supplements, and many others. However, we have found IV vitamin C, and other therapies that impede blood flow or blood vessel development (i.e., angiogenesis blockers), to be incompatible with the concurrent use of the immunometabolic enzymes as they make them less effective. For more detailed information on these finer points, it is likely easiest to contact our offices for further consult.

Overall, more is not always better when it comes to trying to heal the body. It is a fine line to ride between doing enough to "get ahead of the situation" and encourage healing and repair versus overwhelming and/or confusing the body with too many things going on at once. We have seen both possibilities play out in client cases. Sometimes, complications and reactions have happened with clients when they try to do too much at once in terms of other concurrent therapies. I like to use the analogy of a garden to understand that often, time is the oft missing variable in the therapeutic equation. One can have ideal soil, enough sun, enough rain, and just the right temperature to start your garden. But if you sit on the side of your garden and get frustrated that after one week of planting, you don't have a producing garden yet, you're forgetting that the natural world—and our bodies included—have their own schedules and LIMITS to how much can happen in a given time.

While it is important to monitor status and progress during the Kelley protocol with the previously mentioned tests (or with any protocol), we also must not forget to give things time to transform and to not always "throw the whole kitchen sink" at a situation. More is NOT always better, no matter what the protocol.

# CHAPTER NINE

## Quality Matters: A Guide to Relevant Resources, Choosing Quality Products, and the Importance of Quality Supplements

It must be said that the quality of all products, food, supplements, personal care products, and more are paramount for anyone undertaking this program or trying to be healthy (and stay healthy)! Unfortunately, in our hypercapitalistic culture, too often profit trumps safety and quality when it comes to products, and because supplements and especially cosmetics and other personal care items are not tightly regulated for quality and safety, many products can be brought to the market without proper testing and concern for long-term safety with regular use by consumers. As mentioned earlier, only 1% of the approximately 84,000 chemicals used in the marketplace today are tested for long-term safety. That is a scary statistic!

That is why it is so important for consumers, and especially those dealing with serious illness, to learn how to evaluate products carefully for safety and purity, as well to understand the ins and outs of the supplement industry (in the US at least, as it does differ considerably between countries, such as Canada), of how it generally works (both pros and cons), and what to watch out for in general when it comes to understanding supplement formulation, quality, evaluation, and more.

## A Brief Primer on Supplements

Unlike pharmaceutical drugs and the federally controlled stringent testing around active ingredient contents and amounts, etc., supplement quality and testing is largely the responsibility of the manufacturer in the US. Thus, this leads to a vast array of products with varying quality, testing, and standardization. So, it is important whenever considering products that you feel confident about a company's reputation and commitment to quality and research-based formulations. Some companies excel at prioritizing this in their product formulations and manufacturing versus others that are more about price point, and thus, you'll find them more often available at discount retailers.

However, this often means that testing for potency, the quality of formulations, and added ingredients (which we term "excipients") is not as big of a priority, and thus, you can often expect to get inferior products at such places on multiple levels. To some extent, you get what you pay for in the supplement industry, as it takes extra money to pay for third-party testing, investigating the latest research on dosing and optimal types of ingredients, and more to produce a top-tier product.

When you're in doubt about a brand, dosing, or product formulation, we suggest a couple of tips:

I.     *You can request what we call a certificate of analysis on any given product from any quality supplement manufacturer.*

   a. This certificate will be produced by an independent, third-party company that will evaluate the product for potency (i.e., does it actually have the ingredients and amounts as listed on the label or not?), purity (i.e., ensuring there are no bacterial, fungal, or heavy metal contaminations in the ingredients), and other relevant product specifications. If a company doesn't do such testing and/or won't provide such documentation, this is a red flag, and in such a case, it is probably best to look for another source.

II.    *Talk to your qualified, knowledgeable integrative or holistic health practitioner about the brands/ products if in doubt.*

   a. Those who are thoroughly trained and deeply experienced in natural/integrative medicine typically are well versed on supplement companies' reputations in the industry and can likely help you discern if a product is a good and quality choice for you and your needs. They may also have some good ideas on alternative products if they feel that the item you may be asking about is not the best fit for you due to the dose, type of ingredients, or other reasons.

III.   *Become knowledgeable about using medical*

*databases and trustworthy resources for verifying* ingredients, *dosing, etc.*

   a. Most individuals are not aware that there are a multitude of resources on various supplements that are free to access when you're in question over what something does, what might be a typical dose for X, Y, or Z issue, etc. Some of these resources that I'd suggest noting and looking at potentially include:

IV. Medical search engines, such as the National Institutes of Health, PubMed, Google Scholar, and SearchMedica

V. Industry periodicals, such as the Townsend Letter

VI. Resource books such as the *PDR for Nutritional Supplements* and *The Complete German Commission E Monographs* (great for herbal medicine)

This is just a small sampling of some top resources as there are many, many others out there nowadays, but this is a good place to get started when in question or confused.

Supplements that are stocked in practitioner offices and used by experienced natural health care practitioners will generally be of better quality and formulation than what may be commercially available in many common stores that individuals tend to shop in.

Some practitioners have also partnered with online resources/companies, such as Emerson Ecologics, Fullscript, and Natural Health Partners, that have acted as third-party, quality-controlling supplement "brokers" to help patients, near and far, access high-quality supplements. This can be a very helpful way for providers to ensure clients and patients are using better quality products and can readily access them via the internet, no matter where they may be across North America, as such companies will typically ship orders anywhere needed across the US and Canada. Again, remember, Amazon doesn't have such quality control, nor does it have climate control for supplement storage, so beware of going there for many of your supplements!

The products referenced and suggested in this work have undergone similar quality control and have had much focus and attention paid to their quality formulations. For individuals to get optimal results, one must also use and dose quality products accordingly. Thus, the two are intricately dependent upon each other to accomplish optimal health improvements.

## An Essential Note on the Importance of Using the Most Optimal Pancreatic Enzyme Formulation

Fifty years ago, Dr. Kelley talked in interviews about the enormous importance of high amounts of chymotrypsin in the selected pancreatic enzyme formula to ensure the optimal ability of the enzymes to assist the body in helping to break down tumor sites and cells.[62] Yet today, due to the cost and difficulty in manufacturing a product to such specifications, there is only one product, available, through practitioners only, that upholds these particular specifications of chymotrypsin in the respective formulation.[63] Having worked

---

62  Cancer Control Journal, July/August 1973.

63  Other commercially available formulas do not contain nearly the

alongside Dr. Kelley for seven years, Ms. McDougle knew the extreme importance of getting a manufacturer to make the product to such specifications. Thus, she spent a number of years working to find a manufacturer who could meet these stringent requirements. Ultimately, she was able to reliably ensure the manufacturer could produce an extremely potent pancreatic enzyme blend that maintained the desired 84,000–92,000 USP units per capsule in the formula to produce optimal clinical results for clients' greatest benefits.

This is rarely discussed nor known in the larger health community, and yet it is so important when a client or practitioner is considering undertaking the protocol that they use the most appropriate formula to get the most potential benefit. This is the last enzyme formula Dr. Kelley developed and used clinically with Pamela McDougle in the 1990s, and the addition of the chymotrypsin at this noted level was never present in any of the other formulas prior.

**********

The selected listing of items to follow in Chapter 11 are useful references of items that are suggested for use to accomplish key components of this protocol, including the enzymes. Substitutions of such may potentially result in different health influences and outcomes in a given case that are too varied to predict or offer guidance on here.

---

levels of chymotrypsin that this formula does and thus are not advised as an equivalent substitute for a client wishing to undertake the program.

# CHAPTER TEN

## Concluding Thoughts from the Past to the Present, and Hope for the Future

Throughout history, humanity has had a dangerous tendency to get mired down into certain, seemingly "truthful" or "self-evident" perspectives on various issues that we have either too often failed to question enough and/or fought viciously over (even to the death) to protect because it would threaten the status quo. There are MANY such examples from history, but a few include: 1) that the Earth is the center of the universe; 2) that the Earth is flat; 3) and that mental illness is due to "evil spirits." So often, it takes decades, if not generations, for public perspectives and medical opinions to catch up to what research and empirical data tell us.

A substantial part of this, I feel, still relates to the fact that not enough people are being taught the importance of and the skill set of critical thinking and deductive reasoning (and that goes for health care providers too). As both a former student for more than a decade and now an educator, I have seen that it is not being taught in most education programs, and that is negatively affecting us in a multitude of ways, **especially** when we're facing serious medical deliberations. It should be standard practice that we all, providers and patients alike, should be routinely looking at the pros and cons of choices, especially when it comes to medical considerations, by carefully weighing the published evidence and by staying open-minded to more than just such, as it is well known that current research studies are far from perfect, are becoming increasingly difficult to replicate in repeat studies, and are, at times, far from being completely unbiased.[64]

The same goes for existing treatment protocols, which are often slow to evolve and often trapped in vectors of dogma and politics. We should be thinking: What does the research really suggest, and does that make sense biochemically? Physiologically? Circumstantially? What might we want to do differently, even if it isn't "the standard of care," if it really makes sense?

Finally, it's important that we remember and acknowledge that we have not yet thoroughly investigated many, many possibilities when it comes to various therapies and treatments already in existence, let alone not yet developed.

I believe that years from now, individuals will look back at the current paradigm governing typical cancer treatment and widely see it in a similar light, noting just how much of it is short-sighted, outdated, fraught with political agenda, and has much room for improvement. However, for those of us who don't want to wait for such a moment (or can't due to

---

64  https://www.nationalreview.com/2017/11/research-replication-crisis-
    growing-problem/

their health!), the time to act is now to incorporate the many tools and out-of-the-box approaches we already know of to improve our odds in overcoming cancer and improving our nutritional status, detoxification ability, and more.

Dr. Kelley has given us such tools by way of this protocol and illustrated through years of work and dedication that there are other ways to help ourselves recover from chronic illness that, at times, have been deemed impossible by those "in the know."

It is so important that in each individual case, we "dig deeper" into the many roots of dysfunction that are contributing to one's illness. In over a decade and a half of clinical experience, I have seen many patterns in cases seemingly setting the stage for chronic illness to develop, most often as some blend of the following:

- Unaddressed/unresolved emotional traumas

- Latent/ongoing chronic infections

- Chronic gut health problems leading to nutritional deficits and malnutrition

- Toxicity issues from toxicant exposure (from a multitude of sources)

- Chronic sleep problems

- Structural damage and/or injuries due to accidents, falls, and more

- Unaddressed dental issues such as "focal point infections" linked to failed root canals, ill-fitting fillings, etc.

So, while the many things that are presented in this manual

will be incredibly helpful tools and important pieces of the puzzle in helping many individuals, I cannot say they will address all relevant health issues for all people in all cases.

Thus, it is **imperative** for any of you reading this that you go inward and look deeply at what else may be contributing to your state of illness. Sometimes being honest with yourself about such things can be scary, but it is a vital part of this process. Having counseling support in place, if needed, can be vital here in helping support you through this often difficult awakening process. Additionally, it is very important to connect with a qualified integrative or holistic practitioner that can also help you further investigate your situation by way of careful intake, testing, assessment, and follow-up.

You must think of this process as doing "medical detective work"—where every stone needs to be looked at, turned over, and examined for clues. Think of how Sherlock Holmes might investigate a new mystery, for those Sir Arthur Conan Doyle fans out there. So often in medicine, we just skim the surface and see the "tip of the iceberg," whereas in reality, the "heart" of the case is lying deeper beneath the surface.

I believe strongly that if people are well, that if they love themselves and receive love and nourish themselves both physically AND emotionally, we can change the world to be a better, kinder place filled with more possibilities, authenticity, and equity for all. But if you are a prisoner to your health and body, and/or are struggling with some core self-acceptance issues, the vast majority of your energy and life force will be tied up in simply trying to survive, get through the day, and maintain appearances. In traditional Chinese Medicine, so much of illness is linked to blocked, imbalanced, depleted, and suppressed Qi flow. **I've seen this so often in practice over the years in a multitude of cases.**

Our goal, for each and every one of us, should be to thrive on all levels. The notable psychologist Abraham Maslow noted similarly in his groundbreaking "Hierarchy of Needs" pyramid, first proposed way back in 1943. While criticized by some, it has helped to seemingly explain a lot of human needs and the striving to fulfill such, at least in more Western, individual-centered societies.[65] It suggests if we are mired in just trying to meet physiological and safety needs, we will stay in the "basement" or at the bottom of the pyramid, not allowed to progress upward toward full self-actualization and fulfillment of self-esteem needs.

**So with my deepest-seated encouragement, I urge each of you to get up and rise out of the "basement!" Work on your mental, emotional, spiritual, and physical spheres that contribute to the miracle that is you!**

Surrounding yourself with positive people, messages, loving affirmations, and inspiring resources can have profoundly beneficial impacts on our immunity, stress levels, and more.[66] If a religious or spiritual connection in your life has been missing, this may be a wise time to explore connecting to a higher power, whatever this may be for you.

This diagnosis can be very difficult and require much courage to face. Some of you may also need to reckon with deep, big things that you have long since "buried" that are

---

65	https://journals.sagepub.com/doi/10.1177/0022167891313010; https://journals.sagepub.com/doi/abs/10.1177/002216702237123

66	https://journals.sagepub.com/doi/abs/10.1177/0956797610362061; https://onlinelibrary.wiley.com/doi/abs/10.1002/smi.2471

also very frightening. We know this is not an easy process or time to go through. Yet, it must be done.

Thus, given all of this, it is SO IMPORTANT that you get as much support around you as possible so that you are able to face all of this music. Please take this suggestion seriously. It's hard for extra support to be a bad thing, but I have seen time and time again what isolation and lack of support do to negatively impact cases.

But you CAN do it. It is possible.

Dr. Kelley did it.

And many others have as well. So, it is with deep hope and optimism that we leave you as you embark on this new path ahead of you. You are not alone in this journey.

# CHAPTER ELEVEN

## References, Resources, and Links

### Product and Clinician Resources

**Green coffee:** https://sawilsons.com/

**Amino acids:** These are available via www.bodyhealth.com and other sites such as Fullscript.

**High-potency immunometabolic enzymes:** Can be obtained via Visionary Health at www.drericwoodnd. com (1-954-616-8150) or Pamela McDougle's office (see listing below)

**Sauna resources:** https://drlwilson.com/articles/sauna_therapy.htm

**Coffee enema supplies:** McKesson Medical-Surgical: https://mms.mckesson.com/; Seeking Health 1-800- 547-9812: https://www.seekinghealth.com/

**Eliminator II & Selectrolytes:** Health Best Products: 1-208-345-3147

**Dr. Eric Wood, ND, MA and Visionary Health Inc.:** 1-954-616-8150. www.drericwoodnd.com *Consultations on guidance with the protocol, six-month programs, and more information can be obtained by calling the office.*

**American College of Healthcare Sciences:** www.achs. edu

**Pamela McDougle, NC:** 1-208-424-7600. *Consultations on guidance with the protocol and more information can be obtained by calling the office. www.pamelamcdougle.com*

**John Patrick University:** www.jpu.edu

**National University of Healthcare Sciences:** www. nuhs.edu

## Reframing Resources

https://inlpcenter.org/

Tyrrell, Mark. *New Ways of Seeing: The Art of Therapeutic Reframing.* 2014.

https://positivepsychology.com/cbt-cognitive-behavioural-therapy-books/

# Bibliography


https://heilkunst.com/biography.html  http://www.homeoint.org/morrell/articles/pm_miasm.htm

https://www.homeopathycenter.org/homeopathy-today/thought-behind-action-what-are-miasms

https://www.medicalnewstoday.com/articles/288916

https://www.cancer.org/cancer/cancer-basics/lifetime- probability-of-developing-or-dying-from-cancer.html

https://www.cdc.gov/nchs/data/dvs/lead1900_98.pdf

https://www.livescience.com/21213-leading-causes-of-death-in-the-u-s-since-1900-infographic.html

Murray, Michael, and Joseph Pizzorno. *Encyclopedia of Natural Medicine*. Prima Publishing, 1998.

Campion, F. AMA and U.S. Health Policy Since 1940. AMA Publications, 1984.

https://www.ncbi.nlm.nih.gov/pmc/articles/PMC3543812/
https://www.ncbi.nlm.nih.gov/pmc/articles/PMC3241518/

http://www.enzyme-facts.com/enzymes-history

https://www.researchgate.net/publication/5863901_Cancer_is_a_somatic_cell_pregnancy

Beard, J. *The Enzyme Treatment of Cancer*. Chatto and Windus, 1911.

https://www.wobenzym.de/

http://www.organic-systems.org/journal/92/JOS_Volume-9_Number-2_Nov_2014-Swanson-et-al.pdf

https://news.gallup.com/poll/201710/americans-dining-frequency-little-changed-2008.aspx

https://www.ncbi.nlm.nih.gov/pmc/articles/PMC3639863/

https://wholehealthsource.blogspot.com/2011/05/fast-food-weight-gain-and-insulin.html

https://www.healthline.com/nutrition/11-graphs-that-show-what-is-wrong-with-modern-diet#section9

Johnson R.J., et al. Potential Role of Sugar (Fructose) in the Epidemic of Hypertension, Obesity and the Metabolic Syndrome, Diabetes, Kidney Disease, and Cardiovascular Disease. *The American Journal of Clinical Nutrition*, 2007.

https://www.dailymail.co.uk/health/article-6981315/ Millennials-health-plummets-age-27-study-finds.html

https://www.cnbc.com/2018/04/17/how-much-more-expensive-life-is-today-than-it-was-in-1960.html

https://www.uchicagomedicine.org/forefront/news/2006/

july/new-study-shows-people-sleep-even-less-than-they-think-whites-women-and-wealthy-sleep-longer-better

https://www.psychologytoday.com/us/blog/sleepless-in-america/201001/are-we-really-getting-less-sleep-we-did-in-1975

https://articles.mercola.com/sites/articles/archive/2015/07/16/average-american-sleep.aspx

https://www.alternet.org/2015/07/84000-chemicals-use-humanity-only-1-percent-have-been-safely-tested/

https://www.pbs.org/newshour/science/it-could-take-centuries-for-epa-to-test-all-the-unregulated-chemicals-under-a-new-landmark-bill

http://old.iss.it/binary/publ/cont/ANN_08_04%20 Binetti.1209032191.pdf

https://www.ncbi.nlm.nih.gov/pmc/articles/PMC2562028/

https://www.nbcnews.com/health/cancer/50-years-progress-halves-smoking-rate-can-we-reach-zero-n7621

https://www.ewg.org/release/roundup-breakfast-part-2-new-tests-weed-killer-found-all-kids-cereals-sampled

https://www.ewg.org/release/massive-study-finds-eating-organic-slashes-cancer-risks

https://www.ncbi.nlm.nih.gov/pubmed/25789375
https://www.ncbi.nlm.nih.gov/pubmed/15250815/
https://www.ncbi.nlm.nih.gov/pubmed/27347892

https://www.banyanbotanicals.com/info/ayurvedic-living/

living-ayurveda/yoga/nadi-shodhana-pranayama/

https://www.ncbi.nlm.nih.gov/pmc/articles/PMC2724877/

https://www.ncbi.nlm.nih.gov/pubmed/1801007/

https://news.harvard.edu/gazette/story/2002/04/meditation-dramatically-changes-body-temperatures/

https://health.clevelandclinic.org/what-happens-when-your-immune-system-gets-stressed-out/

https://www.sciencedirect.com/science/article/abs/pii/S0165178198001310

https://www.ncbi.nlm.nih.gov/pubmed/9251165?dopt=AbstractPlus

https://time.com/5259602/japanese-forest-bathing/

https://www.psychologytoday.com/us/blog/the-athletes-way/201612/is-shrinking-optimism-tied-drop-in-us-life-expectancy

https://www.independent.co.uk/life-style/health-and-families/optimist-life-span-expectancy-health-benefits-age-study-a9079206.html

https://europepmc.org/article/med/91433 https://jcp.bmj.com/content/49/4/329.abstract

https://www.sciencedirect.com/science/article/pii/S0009912004001274

https://www.tandfonline.com/doi/abs/10.3109/07357909009012053

https://europepmc.org/article/med/8552208

https://www.waterdamagedefense.com/pages/water-damage-by-the-numbers

Stossel, Richard. "The Dangers of Microwave Radiation Cannot Be Ignored." *Natural News and Global Research*, Apr 2, 2011.

Joshi, Amit D., et al. "Meat Intake, Cooking Methods, Dietary Carcinogens, and Colorectal Cancer Risk Findings from the Colorectal Cancer Family Registry." *Cancer Medicine*, 2015.

https://www.ewg.org/foodnews/clean-fifteen.php https://kellybroganmd.com/the-benefits-of-coffee-enemas/

https://health.clevelandclinic.org/hyperthermia-why-heat-can-make-cancer-treatments-more-potent/

https://corporate.dukehealth.org/news-listing/feature-duke-physicians-turn-heat-tumors-hasten-their-demise

http://altmedrev.com/archive/publications/16/3/215.pdf http://drlwilson.com/BOOKS/saunabook.htm.    http://www.ewg.org/skindeep

*Cancer Control Journal*, July/August 1973.

https://www.nationalreview.com/2017/11/research-replication-crisis-growing-problem/

https://journals.sagepub.com/doi/10.1177/0022167891313010

https://journals.sagepub.com/doi/abs/10.1177/002216702237123

https://journals.sagepub.com/doi/abs/10.1177/0956797610362061

https://onlinelibrary.wiley.com/doi/abs/10.1002/smi.2471

Johnson, Steven and Nasha Winters. *Mistletoe and the Emerging Future of Integrative Oncology,* 2021.

# Image Credits

| | |
|---|---|
| Back In My Day | https://www.lendingtree.com/student/millennials-have-it-worse-study/ |
| Sugar Consumption | https://ajcn.nutrition.org/article/S0002-9165(23)13505-2/fulltext |
| Where Americans Eat | https://law.creighton.edu/sites/law.creighton.edu/files/media/Where%20Americans%20Eat.jpg |
| Adoption of GE Crops | https://www.envirogadget.com/wp-content/uploads/2016/07/Eco-Friendly-GMO-3.jpg |
| Number of Children | https://www.countercurrents.org/Autism-and-GMOs.jpg |
| Age Adjusted Deaths | https://www.countercurrents.org/Intestinal-infection-and-GMOs.jpg |
| Major Decline | https://www.bcbs.com/the-health-of-america/reports/the-health-of-millennials |
| The Biotxin Pathway | https://www.survivingmold.com/resources-for-patients/diagnosis/the-biotoxin-pathway |
| Water Damage Defense | https://www.waterdamagedefense.com/pages/water-damage-by-the-numbers |